'Weaving together intel... ...ly the story of mastery but... ...re is much here to inspire,...'
— *Dr Mark J. Langweiler, DC, DAAPM,*
University of South Wales

'Nora Franglen writes with wisdom and heart and touches on the most profound aspects of life. This book is an inspiring and insightful account by an acupuncturist, teacher, and most of all, an ever-searching human being.'
— *Stefanie Sachsenmaier, senior lecturer in Theatre Arts,*
Middlesex University, and Tai Chi practitioner

'The spirit of five element acupuncture chose well when it met Nora Franglen. Nora writes about her life in acupuncture through the window of the elements with genuineness, joy, passion, humility, and a wry sense of humour. This, her seventh book, is not just a masterclass for acupuncturists but also for psychotherapists and indeed any student of human nature.'
— *Jean Ransome, person-centred psychotherapist*

'The art of Chinese medicine, and much of classical Chinese thinking, lies in the subtle observation of things. Nora's many years of acupuncture practice, plus a variety of other life skills, have contributed to making her an expert in the art of observation. This delightful book provides both great pleasure and wise instruction; written more specifically with five element acupuncturists in mind, it can nevertheless be enjoyed equally by practitioners of any kind, and by anyone interested in the observation of life.'
— *Sandra Hill, acupuncturist, co-founder of Monkey Press,*
and author of Chinese Medicine from the Classics

A FIVE ELEMENT LEGACY

From the Five Element Acupuncture *series by Nora Franglen*

Blogging a Five Element Life
ISBN 978 1 84819 371 0
eISBN 978 0 85701 328 6

On Being a Five Element Acupuncturist
ISBN 978 1 84819 236 2
eISBN 978 0 85701 183 1

The Handbook of Five Element Practice
ISBN 978 1 84819 188 4
eISBN 978 0 85701 145 9

Patterns of Practice
Mastering the Art of Five Element Acupuncture
ISBN 978 1 84819 187 7
eISBN 978 0 85701 148 0

Keepers of the Soul
The Five Guardian Elements of Acupuncture
ISBN 978 1 84819 185 3
eISBN 978 0 85701 146 6

The Simple Guide to Five Element Acupuncture
ISBN 978 1 84819 186 0
eISBN 978 0 85701 147 3

A FIVE ELEMENT LEGACY

NORA FRANGLEN

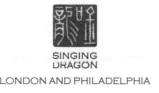

SINGING DRAGON

LONDON AND PHILADELPHIA

First published in 2018
by Singing Dragon
an imprint of Jessica Kingsley Publishers
73 Collier Street
London N1 9BE, UK
and
400 Market Street, Suite 400
Philadelphia, PA 19106, USA

www.singingdragon.com

Library of Congress Cataloging in Publication Data
Names: Franglen, Nora, author.
Title: A five element legacy / Nora Franglen.
Description: London ; Philadelphia : Jessica Kingsley Publishers, 2018.
Identifiers: LCCN 2017059760 | ISBN 9781848194007
Subjects: LCSH: Medicine, Chinese. | Health.
Classification: LCC R602 .F73 2018 | DDC 613--dc23 LC record available at https://lccn.loc.gov/2017059760

British Library Cataloguing in Publication Data
A CIP catalogue record for this book is available from the British Library

ISBN 978 1 84819 400 7
eISBN 978 0 85701 358 3

Printed and bound by CPI Group (UK) Ltd, Croydon, CR0 4YY

For my family

Contents

PART 4: TEACHING OTHER PRACTITIONERS

My Seventh Book

I discovered that, to the Chinese, an 80th birthday is a very auspicious date. My Chinese hosts had been aware of my age ever since my first arrival over there which happened to coincide with my 75th birthday. Each year after that they were keen to remind me with glee of the importance of celebrating my 80th birthday when it eventually arrived in October 2016. So, as my 79th year drew to a close, I was well prepared for something to happen at my next visit, but what I did not expect was to be led into a room filled with all my students, and with a great fanfare to watch a very large birthday cake with candles and 'Happy 80th Birthday' on it being wheeled in by students in traditional dress. And then for other students to sing and dance in front of me, and everybody to give me offerings of small red envelopes, each presented to me and received by me with great joy. It was a lovely way not only to celebrate my birthday, but to be made aware of the warmth with which I am surrounded on each of my many visits to China.

Up to this point I had not really been aware of the passing of each decade, perhaps because I was simply too busy to think about it, but of course each decade represents a new milestone in the direction of life, gaining greater significance with passing time. The celebration surrounding my birthday therefore made me want to assess more clearly what I believed I had achieved in my life and what I had left to achieve, if I am to be granted more time to fulfil what I would like to do. The start of this new decade therefore made me see how important it was for me now to take stock. This, my seventh book, represents my assessment of my life as five element acupuncturist to date.

I have now completed more than 35 years' study of the elements, first as a patient, then as a student, as a novice practitioner, as a teacher of other students and finally now as practitioner and teacher of other teachers – all of those years in the service (and this is not too laden a word) of five element acupuncture, and thus naturally in the service of the five elements which constitute its foundation and the rationale for its very existence. They form the rationale for its persistence, too, for the concept of the five elements is a very ancient concept of what constitutes and creates a human being, what defines the emotions which guide that human being's life, and what shapes the way in which that human being may fall prey to all manner of sicknesses and diseases of the body, and all manner of sadnesses and joys of the soul residing within that body. These 35 years have taught me much about the human being, including a great deal about myself.

Throughout these years my thoughts about myself and thoughts about the human condition have intertwined constantly, as discoveries from my practice have fed into who I am, as practitioner but above all as a human being. I hope in this my 81st year that I have gained some wisdom and put aside some childish things, whilst hoping, too, that the child in me has not been completely absorbed into the adult. Indeed, I often find myself revelling in the ridiculous in a completely new way, allowing myself increasingly to express the side of me which has always been there, that aspect which likes openly to express a joy in life, a joy my Fire element has not always been able to express when at times overburdened. Now, for some reason, probably because I am shuffling closer and closer

each year to the end of my days, it is allowing itself full
rein, doing things and saying things which before it might
not have allowed itself.

I found myself saying to a friend recently that I was
beginning to regard myself as a 'funny old woman', one
of those people encountered in the street who addresses
strangers and mutters to herself. I have not quite yet
reached the muttering stage, but I find myself increasingly
talking to people passing by, with observations on all
manner of things which have caught my eye and are
triggering new thoughts. The sagas of Brexit and Trump,
this year's dominating events, have unleashed in me so
much righteous anger about what this country has voted to
do to itself, that I can scarcely contain my indignation and
sadness, wanting to express them to those whose glances
happen to cross mine in the street or who stand next to
me in a queue. Of course I unashamedly prompt such
discussions because I have proudly worn badges which, on
alternate days, stated either '1 of the 48%' or 'Brexit does
not mean Brexit', open invitations to carry on political
discussions with those close enough to read the messages.

And the heartening thing about the political turmoil
Brexit has unleashed is that it has broken down some
of the walls we build between people. I was reminded of
this today by a small but happy incident in a shop. It was
a lovely Italian paper shop, each object in its display a
temptation for me to buy beautifully coloured piles of
Post-it® notes, hand-produced writing paper, or notebooks
of every size and shape. Mulling over some of the goods,
a woman next to me, observing my anti-Brexit badge,
entered into an impassioned conversation with me, which
ended with her choosing one of the extra badges I always
now carry with me to hand over to anyone showing an
interest in having one (and many do, including, recently,
my bus driver and my newspaper-man). By the time we

had wished each other a good day and a happy new year when it arrived (it was 29 December), I felt reassured, as I have often felt recently, that there are so many of my fellow citizens who feel as strongly as I do that the world is a better place for being united in as many large units as possible, whether United Nations, European Union or other groupings. And definitely that we should remain a United Kingdom, however at odds we now seem to be as our differing constituent countries work out their different agendas. We should not be, as can happen now, so bitterly divided into the Haves of Southern England, the Have-Nots of Wales and the North of England, plus the independent-minded Scots and Northern Irish with their own deep need to remain attached not to England, but to the Europe England seems to have rejected.

I have had many similar heart-warming examples of conversations with strangers to enliven my days.

PART 1

A Lifetime of Five Element Acupuncture

CHAPTER 1

BECOMING A FIVE ELEMENT ACUPUNCTURIST

In all the 35 or more years of my practice as a five element acupuncturist I have never for a moment doubted the profound truth of the fundamental principles underlying that practice, the knowledge that the ancient Chinese concepts of the Dao, yin yang and the five elements were symbols not only for the great forces guiding the universe, but at a much more human level also the energies pouring through us from that universe and creating each one of us, body and soul. When I sat in class on the first day of my acupuncture training, and, appropriately for me personally, heard about the Fire element, with at its centre the Heart official, I remember saying to myself exultingly, 'Yes!', for I seemed for the first time to have heard a language spoken, that of the elements, which explained life to me in a way I could immediately understand.

The three years of my undergraduate training have remained for me a highlight of my life, a time of the greatest discovery, not only of those universal forces flowing through me, which helped explain my amazing reaction to my first treatment, but how these forces could be channelled into offering patients the ability to lead fulfilling lives, true to their individual destinies. I learnt that they could also become so overburdened by stresses too strong for them to deal with by themselves that they could succumb to disease of body or soul. I learnt that the acupuncture needle in the hands of a caring practitioner could become an instrument of healing, offering a therapy devised some thousands of years earlier in ancient China and still miraculously in practice today based on the same ancient principles. These three years were to be dedicated to helping me take my place amongst the ranks of thousands of acupuncturists stretching far back in time. I felt this was an awesome inheritance that I was privileged to share.

It has taken me many years of my own attempts at teaching the principles of five element acupuncture truly to recognise what an extraordinary teacher JR Worsley was, and how inspired he was to work his way from being a novice practitioner in the early 1960s to formulating the principles on which the current huge edifice of five element acupuncture was gradually built up over the years. I regard the course I followed in the 1980s as being a remarkable example of how to distil down to their essentials very complex concepts. Even now, after all these years, I can fault no single aspect of the training I received. In the simplest, most comprehensive way possible we learnt about the elements and their officials, slowly, one after the other. We were given to understand that the qualities of these elements had been handed down since time immemorial in one of the oldest of Chinese medical and philosophical texts, the Neijing Suwen. We learnt to observe the workings of the elements in nature, our assignments taking us outside to observe nature at work during the different seasons, our senses instructed to see, smell, hear and feel what before they might have been too dull to perceive. And, of course, we were helped to see our fellow human beings in different ways, gradually teaching ourselves to recognise the workings of the different elements within each one of us.

This is when I first encountered the concept that for some reason we cannot fathom, so mysterious it is, that each human being has a particularly close relationship to one element. This fact can be seen as constituting the basis of our individuality as human beings, giving to each of us the specific characteristics of one particular element. This mark of individuality singles our species out from any other, except perhaps to a much lesser degree some domestic animals, who any animal lover will say show traces of individual characteristics. JR Worsley called this the element of the causative factor of disease, abbreviated for many years to its two initials, the CF. As its name suggests, this dominant element is the first to weaken under sustained stress, and allow disease to invade. Implicit, though, is the understanding that when it is in balance this particular element is also a power for good, leading us smoothly forward in life towards a future defined by this element. I rather audaciously renamed it the guardian element, a term which echoes that of 'guardian angel'. I see it as something which hovers over us to protect and guide us, and it is my strong belief that this element does indeed take on the role of guardian. Initially I called it this quietly to myself, then I started using the name in my teaching and in my writing, so that now I realise it has been adopted quite generally by other five element practitioners.

This element shapes each of our lives, in a profound sense endowing us with the gift of a personal, unique destiny. Somebody for whom Metal is the dominant element, for example, has their life marked at each point by the characteristic desires and needs of the Metal element. This Metal person's approach to life will differ at a profound level from that of a Fire or a Wood person, each element giving the life it dominates its characteristic qualities. Some characteristics of the other four elements which cluster around it in different degrees of importance will also modify this element's influence to some extent, since we are formed of all five elements. The result of this unique intermingling of the strengths of each element within us will eventually imprint each of us with a unique template of elemental influences, making us who we are and unlike any other. I have called this unique elemental imprint the equivalent in element terms of a unique genetic imprint.

I had proof from my own treatment that the philosophical basis of five element acupuncture was valid and true. My Fire element had responded immediately and powerfully to treatment aimed at strengthening it. I felt that I was 'more myself'. As many of my patients have since told me after successful treatment, I felt that I now 'knew who I was'. Being convinced from evidence in myself that each of us had a dominant element, as students we then had the difficult task of honing senses which had become atrophied over the years. We had to practise looking at the colour of people's skin, smelling their bodies (smelling our own after some stressful physical exercise was a good way to start), listening to their voices, and trying to perceive their emotional needs. All the time we were encouraged to delve deep within ourselves to see the workings of our own element, once this had been diagnosed through our own treatment, hopefully by the most experienced five element acupuncturist of them all, JR Worsley, as many of our students were. I, too, was fortunate to have such a diagnosis during my training, which confirmed my original acupuncturist's diagnosis.

By the time we left the Leamington college after our three years there, we were ready to practise and help others, so straightforward and focused on only the essentials had been our training. During this time I had gone through many periods of self-doubt. 'What makes me think that I am qualified to help others?' 'Have I sufficient emotional maturity to deal appropriately with other people's problems?' At a more basic level, 'Do I have the manual dexterity to manipulate the needles appropriately?' and, more pertinently, and perhaps most importantly for me personally, 'Will I be able to cope with inflicting any pain my needling might cause?' After yet another clumsy attempt at shaping a small moxa cone to the required size, I well remember my tutor telling me that I had to improve this skill quickly if she was to pass me fit to go into the final, clinical year when we were to start treating patients.

I am not naturally very dexterous with my fingers, so I still find it ironic that I have spent the last more than 35 years of my life using them as sensitive instruments of healing. What I did find during my training, though, was that I was absolutely fascinated, and remain it to this day, by the truths lying behind what I was learning. Manual dexterity, or the lack of it in my case, was as nothing compared with the thrill of gradually working out ways to relate to a patient, beginning to perceive the imprint of an element in them, and then helping restore them to health.

Here the first practice diagnosis I carried out at the start of my second year became a catalyst for a change in my approach to what I was doing. As I left the volunteer patient's home on that day after my few hours with her I remember the joyful feeling inside me of at last seeing my life heading in such a worthwhile direction. For somehow I found that I had developed the skill, or perhaps had it already in embryonic form inside me, to enable me to ask the right questions in the right way, and to listen to the answers in the right way so that this woman had felt safe enough to reveal all kinds of things about her life which she said that she had told nobody about before. I acknowledged that my moxa rolling skills left a lot to be desired, and even now I think they are not as good as 35 years' practice should have made them, but my ability to empathise seemed to make up for this.

There was also the beautiful moment during my time with this volunteer patient when I began to see clear signs of the Wood element peeping through what she said and how she was saying it. I realised that I had started to direct my questions in a certain way, attempting to see whether this could confirm the direction towards the Wood element which my questioning seemed to be taking me. And I hoped that it wasn't too soon in the development of my sensory skills for me to think that her voice had the kind of forceful edge which I had been taught was one of Wood's characteristics. I was not yet skilled enough, though, to manage to perceive any particular skin colour or smell any particular smell.

This first encounter with a real live volunteer patient at the start of the second year of my course set me truly on the way, and was a turning point in my training. It became the first time that I realised that I had at last found myself a calling worthy of its name, and that I might begin to be worthy of this calling. Up till then, to the surprise of all the other students in my class, I had not really had a sufficiently high opinion of myself to consider myself to be the right kind of person to be an acupuncturist. Unlike all my fellow students, I found, I had decided to start the course because I was fascinated to learn more about something that had so profoundly altered me. Rather oddly perhaps, actually becoming a practising acupuncturist had been far from my mind. The other students did not seem to share my doubts that they might not be suited for this calling. So to find myself in my second year only then beginning to see where this course was leading me was both a great surprise and a relief. Perhaps after all this was a calling that I was more suited to than I had originally thought.

My progress through the different stages of my learning, from undergraduate through to postgraduate level, was at each phase accompanied by some welcome affirmation of my own qualities that helped me gain increasing confidence in my abilities as acupuncturist. The most heart-warming and overwhelming of these was JR Worsley saying to my advanced training class: 'Watch Nora with her patients. That is how you should do it.' The clapping in the classroom as I returned to it after being observed through a two-way screen handling a very distraught patient of mine stays with me to this day, as a reminder of one of the most moving experiences of my life as an acupuncturist. I felt then that my feet were firmly on a path towards a rewarding future.

CHAPTER 2

THE DIFFERENT PHASES OF MY ACUPUNCTURE LIFE

If I look back at what I have so far achieved in that large part of my life dedicated to acupuncture, what I am most aware of is the extraordinary conjunction of what at first seemed to me to be quite fortuitous happenings which have accompanied the whole of my time in acupuncture, and which taken together have pointed me almost inexorably in the direction of becoming an acupuncturist, and then tethered me firmly there, as though bound to something from which I could no longer free myself, and certainly no longer wished to free myself.

There was an inevitability to the progression from my presence at a party where I met a five element acupuncturist, to deciding to have some treatment from him, a treatment which I was told was for body and spirit. And it was to the word spirit I was drawn. It resonated with some unexpressed need deep inside me, and beckoned me with little resistance on to the treatment couch and my first encounter with the needles.

I was surprised that my acupuncturist was so interested in finding out the details of my life, with all its troubles and joys. Instead of needles in my ear, which I had come to expect from seeing acupuncture on TV, they were gently inserted into my back (an Aggressive Energy drain, of course), followed by some more on my hands before I was free to leave. And this is where I can see with hindsight that that part of my life which was from then on to be lived in the company of acupuncture was blessed from the very start, for I was granted the effects of a first treatment that not many of those I have since treated over the years have been given, an overwhelming, totally unexpected reaction which set my life without warning on a completely new path. For I woke the next morning a completely different person. Something had happened inside me, something I could not explain to myself, but which I knew without any shadow of doubt had changed me in some profound way. It was good for me that I was able to experience in myself confirmation of the efficacy of acupuncture. I had no preconceptions of what treatment might do for me, and I needed some such startling proof in order to jolt me so abruptly and turn my life into quite a new direction.

So what exactly did I experience and how did it convince me that here was something, to me then inexplicable, which I felt I had to get to the bottom of and understand? I was, after all, a doctor's daughter, with my whole life till then steeped in the world of Western medicine, the world of the rational and the scientific. I could find no explanation in this world for the changes I experienced the day after my first treatment. And the very words I used to describe these changes were themselves alien and unfamiliar to me. I told myself that a completely different person had awoken the following morning, somebody I could hardly recognise. It was as though this person had suddenly found herself in a new landscape, one in which she felt as though roots grew out of the ground attaching her to the soil beneath her feet. I remember wanting to take my shoes off and walk on the grass. I felt that I now belonged to a different world, one which I knew I was part of, as though before I had become detached from it and unaware of my connections to it.

I was not then, and never have been, a fanciful person. Thoughts such as these did not come easily to me, and, though almost overwhelmed by the power of the images chasing through my brain, I knew that I was experiencing something profound and true. I felt compelled to follow where this new path seemed to be pointing, so I enrolled swiftly into an acupuncture course in Leamington, for no other reason than because this was where my acupuncturist had studied. And again, the original blessing of encountering acupuncture laid another hand of welcome upon me, for I soon realised that this college was the only place to give me what I so earnestly sought – a new understanding of life and, with it, a new vocation. It led me into the world of the five elements, one imbued with the spirit of JR Worsley, its founder, whom I eventually came to regard as my master. That I should have found myself on the first day of my course walking into a building then dedicated in its entirety to a study of the five elements and their application to the healing of the sick in spirit and body proved yet another fortunate step by offering me a calling which satisfied a great need in me to fulfil myself.

Once having experienced such profound changes in myself, I could not hold myself back from seeking to offer to as many people as I could what I had myself experienced. It was fortunate that the time of my enrolment coincided with what I later came to realise was the late flowering of five element acupuncture's influence in acupuncture education in this country, overlapping as it did with the last years when JR Worsley was still in charge and taught at his college. After qualification there then came the period of my training which I regard as its highlight, my postgraduate work, where I was privileged to sit at the feet of JR Worsley, and to form part of the last postgraduate cohort passing through his hands before his resignation from his Leamington college. I finished my Masters course with him at exactly the time at which his association with the college he had founded came to an abrupt, unhappy end. This was when the hand of modern Chinese acupuncture started to reach over to this country, and to cast its shadow over the traditional forms of acupuncture which were so far being taught here. Amongst other things its effect was to have a negative influence on the British acupuncture establishment's opinion of five element acupuncture. JR Worsley decided to resign from his college because he could not accept the introduction of this form of modern Chinese acupuncture into its training, something he strongly felt would dilute the purity of the five element principles that he had put together so skillfully for many years.

These developments in the world of acupuncture therefore placed my beloved five element acupuncture almost on a collision course with what appeared to have become the consensus of acupuncture opinion in this country at the time. The acupuncture world seemed almost uncritically to welcome the principles of modern Chinese acupuncture, which then started to flood into this country and around the world, and persuaded many to turn away from the traditional form of acupuncture which I practised, consigning it to an inferior role and often removing it altogether from the curriculum of acupuncture colleges. Having understood, as I had learnt to do, that five element acupuncture was a complete discipline in itself, I could not accept a judgement that denied it its rightful place.

This ushered in my decision to fight for the survival of five element acupuncture by founding my own college, the School of Five Element Acupuncture (SOFEA), with active support and encouragement from JR Worsley, leading, on the one hand, to 12 years of rewarding work guiding my students through their three years of study, whilst, with my other hand, fighting off those, often from other acupuncture colleges apparently threatened by my unequivocal support for five element acupuncture, who tried in various ways to oppose the school's right to exist.

At each stage of the many years I have devoted to acupuncture, its peaks and troughs appear to have been accompanied by some often surprising and unexpected events confirming the strong belief I had that my life was destined to follow a course set for it. I remember clearly a dream I had in the midst of the turmoil which engulfed JR Worsley's Leamington college as others there fought hard to try to persuade him to include modern Chinese acupuncture in its curriculum, in defiance of his conviction that this was to dilute the purity of five element acupuncture which his teachings had come to represent. I was absolutely convinced that JR was right to hold out against the tide threatening to engulf five element acupuncture, one of the very few he told me who were, but I was unsure what my role in supporting him should be. I was then in the final year of my advanced postgraduate studies with him. I had a flourishing, very satisfying practice working from my home in London, and I had started to hold regular supervisory sessions for Leamington students, at one of which a student said, 'I have learnt more from you in one day, Nora, than I think I learnt at Leamington in a year,' a flattering if untrue remark, but one which resonated with me because it set me wondering whether I should start thinking about teaching in a more structured way.

Then I had this dream, only one of a few which have made such a profound impression on me that I can still remember it clearly with a shiver of excitement. For in this dream JR was standing at the doorway of his Leamington college, surrounded by his staff who were telling me quite vehemently that they were rejecting me as a tutor. JR, however, was quite silent, and simply pointed me away into the distance. The next scene in the dream was of Piccadilly Circus, in the centre of London. Encouraged by the students I had been working with, I had begun to think of setting up a five element college of my own as a way of countering the, for me, devastating developments which had forced JR to resign. I had started looking for premises in London, the first being at a school of osteopathy in central London, only a few minutes from the Piccadilly Circus to which JR had pointed me in my dream. I was quite sure the dream was telling me that JR was encouraging me to have the courage to strike out on my own and that he would be offering me his support.

I didn't realise it at the time, but with hindsight I have become increasingly aware that it must have taken courage to do what I did: I embarked upon a big adventure, setting off on my own to establish a teaching college without any qualifications for doing this, apart from my few years of practice, a few years giving evening classes on five element acupuncture in London and my deeply held conviction that I had to do something to keep the spirit of five element acupuncture alive in an increasingly hostile environment. Nobody else seemed to be as concerned as I was that JR Worsley had felt that he been forced out of the college he had founded and so lovingly tended for 30 years or more, and I was surprised to hear no howls of protest from the many five element acupuncturists he had trained there. Perhaps this was because many acupuncturists may not have known the reasons for his resignation, since acupuncturists can lead quite isolated lives, alone with their patients and dotted around the UK and further afield, and might have been unaware of the political ramifications of the entry of Chinese-promoted traditional Chinese medicine (TCM) into the acupuncture world of this country. Or, I have since thought, perhaps many were simply daunted by the thought of treading in JR's giant footsteps.

The 12 years during which I fought to keep the spirit of five element alive as a stand-alone discipline took their toll on me, finally coinciding with the financial problems caused by the credit crunch, which made me foresee problems in recruiting enough students to justify keeping the school open. The decision to close in 2007 was forced upon me by a threatened sharp rise in our rent as well as some unhappy internal squabbles within my faculty who were not as convinced as I was that I was fighting the right battles. So then there came the downsizing from a large old Victorian factory in Camden Town to a single practice room in Harley Street, from which I continued both to practise and to run postgraduate seminars, extending these to travels to various European countries, and culminating in yet another surprising development, the start of my visits to China. This originated in a quite unforeseen encounter with a Chinese acupuncturist now living in the Netherlands, her enthusiasm for five element acupuncture leading through a few twists and turns directly to my being invited to China, and setting me on to a different, more internationally-based path.

All this time I was adding to my teaching and my practice by writing books, initially to help my students, and then gradually to develop my own ideas, so that now there are six of these out there, with this, my seventh, now being published here. Here my visits to China also opened the door to having my books translated into Mandarin, with the phenomenal numbers sold over there (25,000 at the last count) being testimony to the extraordinary degree of interest sparked by the arrival of five element acupuncture back on its shores.

A great master of any discipline always casts huge sha-dows over any successors. Interestingly, though, far from daunting me, as some have told me it might have, it has actually stimulated me to feel that I am indeed following where JR led, and have always felt that the shadow he cast over me as one of his acupuncture disciples was a kind and encouraging one. I did not feel I needed courage to do what I did in founding SOFEA. Instead, I regarded it as my homage to what I had been taught, and still do. All that I have done since my first days setting up SOFEA, in my practice and in my subsequent postgraduate work, and finally extending this to my current work in China, forms part of a continuing process of homage to someone who had the vision to understand the relevance of this profound form of healing to a modern world, and then had the courage to put this vision into practice.

CHAPTER 3

STARTING TO TEACH

I often wonder how I had the audacity to think that I was in any way qualified even to dream of teaching five element acupuncture, let alone founding an acupuncture college, or that I had the courage to put my plans into practice, as I did, very rashly in my accountant's opinion. The School of Five Element Acupuncture (SOFEA) opened its doors in 1995 as a privately-funded college, independent of any association with a university. I had been in practice for not much more than seven years, and the only teaching I had ever done was in the evening classes I had started to give. It was the success of these evening classes that strengthened my resolve, and made me think that I had something to offer others, particularly my enthusiasm about this new-found calling of mine as five element acupuncturist.

I credit my desire to found a five element acupuncture college to what I learnt during these classes. Like many things in my acupuncture life, including now my intro-duction to China, there seem to have been all kinds of, at first sight, fortuitous events which at the time did not seem very significant, but which later proved to be major turning points in my life. I have already mentioned one of these, the party at which I met a five element acupuncturist. Another one was the fact that a good friend of mine was in charge of organising evening classes at one of the large London evening class institutes, Morley College. She was looking around for interesting new courses to include in her list of classes, and wondered whether I would be interested in talking about acupuncture. At the time, this was an unknown topic for most people, and there were no classes relating to any form of alternative medicine for the lay person to go to. I therefore found myself a pioneer in the field.

At first I hesitated to accept my friend's offer. I had only just qualified, was in the very early stages of my practice and was very unsure as to what I had in me to teach. I remember asking my tutor at Leamington whether it was too early for me to give these talks. His reply was, 'They have asked you, Nora. Do it!' In a similar vein, many years later, when I admitted to JR Worsley that I often felt that I did not know enough to teach my undergraduates, he said, 'You know more than they do', something that I have repeatedly passed on to others worried about their own qualification to teach.

Despite my initial fears, I very soon relaxed into the comfortable atmosphere of a very interested, inter-esting and disparate group of people who had come to listen and learn. As my confidence grew, I spread further afield and gave seminars to several groups of people at different evening classes in London, at one point running three different courses a week, each course consisting of a two-hour talk about the elements for up to ten weeks at a time. What did I talk about? Well, almost exclusively about the elements, and almost never, I later realised, about the actual practice of acupuncture. The needles and the acupuncture points faded into the background, and my thoughts on the elements came to the fore. Classes were fascinated by what they heard, and we talked together at length about how the different elements affected us in our personal lives or at work, leading to many interesting discussions about life in general. I was flattered when I was told at the end of one such series of classes that seven of the participants had decided to apply to the Leamington college to study acupuncture.

Being thrown into the deep end in this way had two profound effects, which have since shaped the rest of my acupuncture career. The first was that I was absolutely free to say what I wanted about the elements, and therefore to develop my own thoughts, without being hampered in any way by what others thought. That allowed me to expand my understanding in unexpected ways, something I realised when I returned to Leamington two years later to start my Bachelor of Acupuncture studies. I became aware then that I had often gone off at a tangent from the generally accepted views of my fellow practitioners. Like a scientist working on their own in their private laboratory, I had done my own experiments without realising this, and come up with my own original answers which often surprised or even shocked others in the class, who had, I felt, often remained rather stuck in the groove carved out for them during their initial training.

I don't think it was arrogant of me to think this. Something similar will always happen when a person works on their own, and their new ideas are not tempered by setting them against what others believe. It was by accepting that I had apparently forged my own individual and rather idiosyncratic five element path, and not been frightened to do this, that I took the first step on the road to where I am now. This forced me to be unafraid of saying and thinking things that others baulked at or considered to be either opinionated or diverging too far from what they had themselves been taught. Interestingly, I never felt that JR Worsley thought this. Indeed, I felt that he actively encouraged my often independent thoughts, giving me the strong feeling that he supported the direction of my thinking on the elements.

The second effect of being cast adrift on my own to do my own teaching without reference to anybody else led to my discovery that I had great delight in passing on my knowledge wherever I could. There was something within me that compelled me to try to hand on to others what I was myself learning. This strengthened my resolve to found an acupuncture college, and has stayed with me increasingly throughout my life as a five element practitioner and teacher.

It also led directly to my starting to have the urge to write. I was prompted to do this first by a publisher who asked me to write one of his series of little books called Simple Guides, this one on five element acupuncture. This was followed by the need to give my students a textbook, which turned into my *Handbook of Five Element Practice*, now expanded in its second edition to include a Teach-Yourself Manual. This addition was prompted by my teaching in China, where I soon realised that very few of my students there would have the opportunity to study with a five element practitioner as I had done during my training. The Handbook was followed in fairly quick succession by four more of my books – *The Keepers of the Soul: The Five Guardian Elements of Acupuncture, Patterns of Practice, On Being a Five Element Acupuncturist* and *Blogging a Five Element Life* – the last two being selections of my blogs since 2011.

All these books have already been or are in the process of being translated into Mandarin to satisfy the overwhelming need for five element writings over there. Since some 25,000 copies of the Mandarin translation of my Handbook have now been sold in the five years since its publication in China, the chances are that the Chinese editions of my other books will sell equally well, helping to spread the word about five element acupuncture to every corner of its vast homeland, China.

The path from my first evening class, as I stood trembling in front of a group of about 20 people, plumbers, secretaries, the unemployed and the retired, all fascinated by what the elements taught them about life and about themselves, to today's Chinese seminars, each time given to over 100 people, with lectures at traditional medicine institutes with audiences of about 500, has been surprisingly smooth, if looked at from the widest perspective. I stumbled many times, particularly as I fought for the right to teach my SOFEA students five element acupuncture in all its purity, and encountered at times what could almost be considered verbal abuse and overt aggression as part of this fight. But looking back, the trajectory was very clear, leading me to where I am now, in the later years of my life. I am privileged to be regarded as an experienced elder statesperson in the acupuncture world, a beacon for five element acupuncture wherever I teach. I am able to forget the unpleasant hurdles which were put in my way, and like to think of myself as having reached sunny uplands, with a wide panorama spread before me, showing me thousands of acupuncturists as enthused as I have been with the beauty and purity of five element practice. Viewed from this standpoint I have been very fortunate to have reached such a high point at this stage in my life.

CHAPTER 4

DIFFICULTIES IN RUNNING A COLLEGE

Apart from the obvious hurdle of actually having the courage to invest my own personal money into founding the school, I had to overcome many practical difficulties. I had no administrative experience at all apart from running a home, working for a few years at the British Council and contributing to the family finances by doing freelance translation work during the day or in the evenings, when the children were in bed. All this was very much part-time working, and was very little suited to giving me the skills I found I needed to set up a school, find the right premises, attract students to it and employ some good tutors. Most important of all, and most time consuming, I had to devise a curriculum from scratch which satisfied my desire to replicate what I had myself been taught, and also, increasingly importantly, which met the ever-expanding requirements of the newly established British Acupuncture Accreditation Board.

The only subjects I had been good at in school were languages. I found I had a gift for these, whilst I had none at all for any scientific subjects, and I could not understand maths. Algebra and geometry were totally alien concepts which I never got to grips with. Languages, however, were something that I seemed to be able to learn surprisingly easily and quickly, and I would soon find myself at home in any foreign language I learned. It is therefore a great sadness to me that I came too late to the one language of

use to me today, Mandarin. It requires the kind of intensive
learning which somebody of my age can no longer apply,
and, linguist that I was, it is one of my greatest regrets that
I did not start learning it when I could have done thirty
years ago when my memory would have been retentive
enough for this most complex of languages.

But since learning and speaking languages appeared
to be my only skill, this was what I studied at university,
and therefore what I continued to use in my working life
afterwards. A modern languages degree in itself was of
little help in setting up my college though. However, what
helped me, I soon realised, were the years of disciplined
work inculcated into me from junior school onwards.
Those were the days when children were not exactly 'seen
but not heard' but were still very much expected to obey
authority in whatever form it took. From standing up as a
teacher came into the classroom, chanting 'Good morning,
Miss' to sitting obediently in rows often silently, listening to
what our teachers taught us, we did what we were told, and
God forbid if we infringed some rule, for then we found
ourselves trembling with fear outside the Headmistress's
study. That fear was enough to keep the school in order.
I can't remember a single disruptive session during lessons.
We listened, we did our homework and seemed to
understand what we learnt, and this way of learning taught
us above all the discipline which has stood me in good stead
ever since, particularly at the time of my metamorphosis
into becoming a principal of an acupuncture school.

We are all shaped by our families and the years of our
education, and we can never shrug these influences off.
Looking back with the hindsight of the years and of the
many happenings in my life, I realise that without this
by now innate sense of the importance of discipline I
would not have been able to achieve what I did. At the
most basic level, somebody running a school and being

responsible for the students' learning for which they were paying me had to have the necessary discipline simply to turn up on time, open up the school, turn on the heating, answer the waiting phone calls, ensure that the right tutor had arrived in time for any specific class, ensure that that tutor had been primed in sufficient time about whatever administrative arrangements were needed on the day (the time of breaks during teaching hour, the start and end times of the day, the homework assignments to be collected and others handed back, problems with a particular student to be addressed), and on and on the list goes. To ensure the successful running of a course required a high degree of disciplined organising ability, added to what I found to be an essential ingredient: the flexibility to cope with the unexpected and take it in my stride.

The problem for me, related to my natural sense that students, too, needed to show a reasonable degree of discipline, was that I failed to take into account the very different educational approaches of my students, all invariably younger than me, or indeed much younger, and therefore growing up in a completely different educational environment, one which allowed for much greater latitude for the students. This I understood only gradually. I was fortunate to have as a near-neighbour a very senior retired tutor of social workers, and she very kindly granted me much time of an evening, when I would return often somewhat disheartened by events at the school. Together we would go through the day's events and she would adroitly point out to me various weaknesses in my approach both to other tutors and to students, which had probably contributed to some difficult moments for me and made me doubt whether I was up to the very heavy task I had set myself of guiding these students towards a professional qualification.

I began to see through what she pointed out to me that I had, to my surprise, a rather authoritarian streak in me which came to the fore when I was unsure how to proceed, and which certainly contributed to some unnecessary friction between me and some students, and sometimes, too, between me and some tutors. It is a regret to me that I only truly learnt to curb this tendency when it was almost too late, and I was close to taking the decision to close the school. Hindsight is always a fine thing, I know, but looking back I realise I would have been a lot happier and run a more successful school if I had learnt earlier that being authoritarian was the absolute opposite of exercising an appropriate level of authority.

What my neighbour did successfully teach me, though, was a lesson that stood me in very good stead during the years of the school, and has continued to stand me in good stead ever since. This was that there was nothing I did which could not in some way be countermanded or offset, no ill-advised action which could not be rescinded or at least have its effect softened. So if I made some mistake by handling a problem with a staff member or a student in the wrong way, I should always be able to mitigate the effects of any clumsy actions I might have taken, of which there were quite a few due to my inexperience.

I always found it difficult, however, to accept un-disciplined behaviour on the part of a student which disturbed other students, such as a student's late arrival which interrupted the others in the class. It continued to irritate me that students who lived nearest to the school in London tended often to be the ones arriving late, whilst those flying in from abroad invariably turned up on time. I am sure that I could have dealt better than I did with this, but I am surprised that I managed 12 years of dealing with such apparently trivial events, when all I wanted to do was help students glory in the profound truths I saw in five element acupuncture.

CHAPTER 5

TEACHING FIVE ELEMENT ACUPUNCTURE

I have been noticing that my approach to teaching is now beginning to take on another shape. I have started to see that what I have set in place in this country, in various European countries and particularly now to a much greater extent in China, demands of me different kinds of approaches, and not simply that of replicating the way I was taught. Here my experiences in China have undoubtedly come to my aid, because to my surprise the Chinese, who may have received only a fraction of the five element training of their Western counterparts, and base themselves on only a paltry few weeks' seminars a year with us, have taken to five element acupuncture 'like ducks to the water', as the saying goes. I realise that this openness to a totally new experience of acupuncture has much to do with a cultural inheritance stretching back thousands of years, which still continues to underpin all aspects of everyday life. Introducing five element acupuncture back into this culture is as though I am opening a door upon a familiar landscape. This is so different from what happens in the West, where students have first to familiarise themselves with totally new concepts.

Taking account of these different cultural heritages raises questions as to the need to work out different ways of teaching five element acupuncture. The culture prevailing in the countries where students learn will demand different approaches, depending on students' familiarity with the

core philosophical concepts underlying traditional acupuncture. The Western model I was brought up with,
and which I carried on teaching at my own acupuncture
college, the School of Five Element Acupuncture
(SOFEA), was based on the conventional structure of a
three-year university-type course. This model does not,
however, suit all circumstances, and certainly not those
I encounter in China. It is quite clear that what a three-
year course can cover is going to be quite different from a
course which extends over only a few weeks a year. What
has surprised me, though, is how quickly my Chinese
students have learnt to adapt their previous clinical
practice to the demands of five element acupuncture
which differ so greatly from the TCM principles they have
learnt. This in turn has made me look more carefully at the
assumptions underlying the standard three-year courses
run by acupuncture colleges in this country.

What exactly do we cover during these three years?
When I started SOFEA, I took as a model exactly what
my training at JR Worsley's Leamington college had
covered. In Year 1 we were introduced to the philosophical
principles underlying all Chinese thought, and their
application to traditional medicine, and studied sufficient
anatomy to locate all acupuncture points. We spent a great
deal of time learning about each of the five elements and
their 12 officials, and were told to observe them in nature
outside as they create the cadence of the seasons. We also
started to observe the actions of the elements within
ourselves and in everybody we encountered.

By the second year we began to put what we had learnt
into practice, carrying out a number of practice diagnoses
on volunteer patients. It was at this point that I suddenly
realised I was embarking upon something I could now
regard as a calling for myself. For the whole of my first
year it had felt as though I was almost sleepwalking into

acupuncture, seeing my time at the college as an interesting episode in an otherwise full life. I had only decided to study it because I was intensely curious to understand a discipline which had had such a profound effect on me. Initially I had no intention of practising it, something that was possible in those early days of acupuncture education, because not only was it relatively easy to pay for the course compared with the fees now charged, but the course itself was spread over far fewer days a year (a weekend every month, if I recall it correctly), and so could easily be integrated into a working life. Applications were also encouraged from people with very little formal education, unlike the need for A-level standards for applicants now, because the emphasis was much more on a person's ability to show compassion for people, rather than on book learning. In fact book learning was positively frowned upon, since JR told us to throw away our books and learn from nature. We were to become 'instruments of nature', and this is how we regarded ourselves.

The final third year was an almost exclusively clinical year during which we had to treat a certain number of patients, and observe the treatments of all the other students studying with us. The course was now weekly, because of the frequent treatments our patients required, and I found myself driving the two hours up the motorway from London early each Saturday morning, often accompanied by a London-based patient. We were only allowed to graduate when we had completed the required number of clinical hours, but also had satisfied our tutors that we were able to deal with the many emotional problems patients faced us with.

In my own training, therefore, we spent much of the three years concentrating on trying to detect the presence of the elements in everybody we encountered, and this included being encouraged to watch as much TV as possible as part of the development of our diagnostic skills. The total number of hours we spent doing this came to many hundreds over the three years of our training. Compare this to what I can offer our Chinese students now, or what any TCM practitioner venturing into the area of five element acupuncture has to accept.

We were therefore fortunate in having the opportunity to spend these three years of our course steeping ourselves in the elements, something Chinese practitioners deeply envy us for. They have to make do with only the few weeks of seminars we give each year, but supplement these with the enthusiasm with which they carry on studying on their own or in groups to add to what we offer them. As there are so few of us who are teaching them, there is no alternative, except to encourage them to develop a mindset in which they start to see themselves as pioneers. Those seeking to learn a discipline like five element acupuncture must therefore now learn to regard themselves as following in the footsteps of JR Worsley and his small band of fellow seekers after acupuncture truths, who had to make do with very little tuition and did most of their learning by themselves. The rest of the time this group had to rely on themselves, as they dispersed to various parts of the country and developed their own approach to what they were learning, each with a different emphasis, but all basing themselves on traditional principles. JR Worsley set up a college in his home town, Leamington Spa, Mary Austin another college in Central London, and Dick van Buren founded the International College of Oriental Medicine (ICOM), still a teaching institute in East Grinstead, Sussex.

To learn more about traditional acupuncture's route of transmission from East to West, it is important to read the excellent book by Peter Eckman, *In the Footsteps of the Yellow Emperor: Tracing the History of Traditional*

Acupuncture.[1] This is the only book I know of which describes the history of this transmission in great detail, with particular emphasis on five element acupuncture.

In a way it could be said that those early seekers after acupuncture based their learning on the well-established and much to be admired principle of the master/pupil relationship, an age-old discipline in which a tradition is passed on by personal transmission from a master to a pupil, who will in turn develop mastery and carry on the transmission to yet another generation. To me, this has always seemed to be the most highly desirable form of learning, but is only possible in cultures where the disciple will be encouraged by their family to hand themselves over entirely to the pursuit of a discipline. This holds true in very few countries now, and only continues to exist in this form mainly in relation to some religious disciplines. It has the obvious disadvantage that very few now have the leisure needed to spend years at the feet of a master, something considered to be entirely appropriate in former times.

Chinese students of five element acupuncture have the advantage over my Western students of inheriting a tradition in which they learn unquestioningly to accept the authority of a master, and where mastery is a designation quite frequently awarded to anybody with sufficient years of experience. I, too, have had to accept that this is how they view me. At first I was very reluctant to take on this role, but soon came to realise that five element acupuncture would lose some of its value in their eyes unless I did. The tradition which they saw me as representing requires that it should be firmly grounded in an inheritance which acknowledges the contribution

1   Eckman, P. (1996) *In the Footsteps of the Yellow Emperor: Tracing the History of Traditional Acupuncture.* San Francisco, CA: Long River Press.

through the ages of a line of masters. I could only claim one master, JR Worsley, which was easy for me to do, since he was acknowledged as such not only by me but by all five element acupuncturists around the world. And thus, being his pupil, I have had to step into the role demanded of me, so that now, lining the walls of wherever I teach, are photos first of JR Worsley, then of me, followed by those of Guy Caplan and Mei Long, my teaching assistants. A tradition without evidence of a progression of this kind would be devalued in the eyes of the Chinese. This helps explain why efforts have been made to connect some of JR's teachings, which he was known to have taken from Japanese acupuncture masters, to a line of traditional Chinese medicine practitioners in Manchuria, which it was thought had found its way from China to Japan at the time of the Japanese invasion. Whether this is historically true or not is not as important to the Chinese as the need to root five element acupuncture as far back as possible in the past, thus further establishing its historical validity.

Faced as I am with what could be seen as the limitations of the five element teaching experience available to my Chinese students, I have had to learn to adapt how I teach to what is possible in the time available, hoping that the enthusiasm and willingness to learn shown will help make up for the obvious lack of time I can dedicate to them. And from the evidence so far this is luckily what is happening. In fact, this enthusiasm can seem to me to outweigh the obvious disadvantages of how little time I can spend with them. I know that in their meetings when I am not there they make constant use of all the video material of my teachings that they have painstakingly collected together over the six years of our visits. I cannot recall a day when a video camera wasn't whirring in front of our faces, either recording every word we said or trailing from practice room to practice room as we treated patients.

This recorded material is now a very active source of learning for everybody, and the various types of social media which students and practitioners sign up to make this much simpler than it would have been years ago, as all our teachings are now widely available to anybody throughout China.

One major difference between Chinese and Western learning attitudes which is also helpful is Chinese students' uncritical acceptance of what they are taught, a discipline no doubt instilled in them by the educational systems they are brought up in. This contrasts with the more free-thinking approach to learning much encouraged by modern Western educational precepts. In one respect, of course, this makes teaching apparently much easier for tutors in China than in the West, because they face less obviously overt challenges from students. The Western approach of encouraging students to question what they are taught as part of their development as curious individuals is something more or less unknown in the Chinese students I have taught. On the other hand, the willingness to learn and the hunger for new forms of learning undoubtedly adds to the Chinese experience, and I suspect that the more questioning Western attitudes will soon become more widespread as Western influences spread and the internet and social media start to draw us all into a common pool of humanity

CHAPTER 6

AN ACUPUNCTURIST'S INHERITANCE

One of the problems with working in an age-old tradition such as ours is that, unlike Western medicine, which has only a few hundred years behind it, we are encumbered by it and privileged to be heirs to it both at the same time, and we often confuse what is a burden of the past with what is its welcome inheritance. The line between the two is not finely drawn, since traditions can always both inhibit and enhance, and a conviction of where the one thing becomes the other will vary depending on the standpoint from which both are viewed.

Perhaps it is that we so revel in what we regard, quite rightly, as our awesome acupuncture inheritance, that we tend to swallow it whole, not pausing to examine which parts of it remain alive to us here in the 21st century and which have died either a lingering death or by swift execution, many centuries ago. With such a long drawn-out tradition trailing behind us, it is very difficult for the non-historian of acupuncture, and I count myself definitely in this category, even to find the time to do more than accept on trust much that we were taught during our initial first training, and with any luck have added to it a little by subsequent reading or learning. And where can you start to learn about two and a half thousand years of your history, except by accepting as true the words of those few industrious souls out there who have acquired the skill and found the time (and time always means money) to explore our inheritance? Often, too, this exploration is not done at the clinical rock face, but at a more generalised level where wider perspectives can be gained, but the clinical ramifications may become lost. And thus there is often a gap between what can be seen as being clinically relevant and what is historically or philosophically of interest, and into that gap much confusion can creep.

And this ancient inheritance of ours is primarily in a language or languages other than our own, and often in an archaic form or many archaic forms of that language as well. So now in addition to becoming historians we have to become linguists! But linguists of a dead language in the case of much of the original material we have inherited. And the interpretation of all dead languages is much open to debate, for we interpret through the prism of the present, with our own modes of thought and expression covering all that we translate with a patina the words and symbols we decipher may never have had. As a translator in a former guise, and a translator of living languages learned from study in the countries which speak them, I know that even the most apparently innocuous phrase can have a nuance in its original expression which its translated words lack. This was one of the reasons why I, a passionate lover of literature, turned to translating more practical technical texts as often providing a more exact one-to-one match of words, leaving the field of my beloved literature to those who did not appear to mind, as I did, that no English word could be found to echo the beautiful phrases I was reading, and to paraphrase them, to me, smacked of a kind of destruction of the very beauty inherent in the originals.

Of course I cannot be too purist, for I have to read in translation all those works whose languages I am not familiar with, but I always read them with these reservations in mind, and nowhere more so than in relation to the great mass of ancient Chinese texts piled up beneath our feet, upon which we make so many attempts, often futilely, I think, to find a modern foothold in ways those ancient writers of old would not, I suspect, have recognised. It often seems to me as though, with our modern feet, we are trying to find a path through some ancient forest along which we must feel our way forward often over the skeletons of dead trees, looking for what is still living amongst so much growth, as hardy survivors from those ancient of days. But how many of such survivors are there? Or how many have changed or mutated over the years almost out of recognition? How many are we attempting to preserve, fossil-like, though long past being of use to us? Of the life still there in this forest I have no doubt at all, for the many successes in my practice confirm this to me, but which trees are still alive and which have decayed long before is often unclear.

There is a danger in this, too, that of adhering too closely to what the past has accepted, which prevents us from venturing out on to new ground. This was not a risk faced by the early pioneers of Western acupuncture, because they had to work out, each in their own way, their own re-interpretation of what they were learning. They needed to do this, because the amount of teaching available to them was strictly limited, and thus they had to spend much time in between exploring different avenues unchallenged and unsupervised. This led directly to the creation of different branches of Western acupuncture. Thus Dick van Buren was pulled towards investigating the world of stems and branches and JR Worsley the world of the elements as expressions of individuality, what he called the causative factors of imbalance. In turn, I, inheritor of this approach, have gone on to call them guardian elements, as others have called them constitutional elements. No doubt there are others waiting in the wings, who will go on to develop their own personal understanding of a particular aspect of acupuncture, which they will in turn hand on to other students, and I sincerely hope that I will prove right in this. And thus the tree grows from branch to branch.

Because all routes of transmission of knowledge are complex and interlinked in often differing and contradictory ways, particularly knowledge such as that on which acupuncture is based, which spans not only centuries but millennia, we are often reluctant to give credence to those areas of our inheritance which lie somewhat outside the narrow boundaries of our own particular small circle of inherited knowledge. Very few of us appear to have enough confidence in our own judgement to allow other people their diverging opinions and not be thrown off-balance by them. It seems to be of importance to us to try to persuade these others that what they believe in is wrong or mistaken, whilst insisting on the appropriateness of our beliefs. Just as we were told when I was younger that it was impolite to get into an argument with other people about either politics or religion, so now I could add acupuncture to my list. It is surprising how vehemently sides are taken, as the adherents of one school or another advance what they consider unassailable claims for their particular branch of acupuncture or for specific techniques or point selections. I suppose the same is true of all disciplines, for I remember that when I told my sister, a psychotherapist, of the divisions in the acupuncture world, she said, 'You should see how psychotherapists behave!' Perhaps we would all like to feel that the secret of our discipline lies in our hands alone, like the acquisition of some esoteric form of knowledge to which only a few initiates, a select band of the chosen few, amongst them, of course, ourselves, hold the key, and that all those who think or act differently have somehow got it wrong.

I used to be as guilty of such blind prejudices as everybody else, for prejudices they surely were, until I started running courses for non-five element acupuncturists, and realised how much more we had in common than I had previously thought. And their surprise was matched by mine. What I found was that, by dwelling first on what we had in common, when the moment came to move on to those areas of our practice which we did not have in common it was as though we were simply moving on to a less familiar acupuncture landscape, rather than on to totally alien territory. It also soon became clear to me that the essential foundation to all the different practices we were engaged in was our own strong confidence that what we were offering our patients stemmed from a discipline that was what I call true. In other words, that it had a valid claim to do what it said it was doing. If it achieves results, then it can be called a valid discipline, and be counted as one of the many ways in which a human being can be helped back to health and balance. If it does not, then we must query its legitimacy.

In some ways, it is interesting for me to note that over the years I have worked to some extent backwards, in time as well as in thought – in time, from a purely practical acupuncture as I practise it now back to what underpins it, as though through the branches back down to the trunk and to the root. I realise, too, more than I did previously, I think, that, provided I am sitting on a living, healthy branch, the root is always there below me, sending up sap to revitalise all that I do, however hidden to me is often this passage of transmission of knowledge. I am now encouraged to look at what I do from a somewhat different angle, one of greater curiosity, but also one of trying to determine whether what I do is based only on a kind of hearsay, on what others have told me, or on what I have myself proven to myself is effective. In other words, have I any proof from my own practice that what I have learnt is true? It may seem odd for me, at this advanced stage in my practice, to query what I do in this way, but there is very little evidence that acupuncturists are engaged in any depth in such enquiry, as I certainly was not in the early days of my practice.

This is understandable, of course, because it is in the nature of all learning that we have to take most, if not nearly all of it, on trust. We can't, as it were, re-invent the wheel every time we lift a needle. We have to some extent to accept that others before us, in acupuncture's case often many centuries before us, have based their acquisition of knowledge on their own clinical experiences, and to hope that it is this proof from clinical, rather than theoretical, experience that has been handed down as our inheritance.

Of course with time, and over the long period of time we are dealing with here, some, if not much, of this accrued learning will be found to have either lost its relevance for a more modern age or be revealed to have been false in the first place. Here I need only point to those long lists of associations with the elements (planets, grains, animals, etc.) which are no longer learnt by students, let alone used clinically, but which formed the bedrock of past learning. Does a particular planet or animal have a particular resonance for a given element or not? Has anybody researched this in any way? It is indeed difficult to see how evidence for or against such correspondences could be collected. What we are left with from these long lists are some, a very few only, which are clinically valid, and proven to be so from current clinical practice, such as, in the case of five element acupuncture, the sensory associations of colour, sound, smell and emotion which form the mantra of the five element acupuncturist of today. These I know from my own and others' practice to have proven clinical validity. Many more of these lists of associations lie buried in old books gathering dust on library shelves, of interest only because they point to an earlier time when a worldview dominated in which all things were related to one another symbolically as a way of lessening the fears the world and its happenings aroused.

I do not feel that acupuncturists have in any way so far properly examined the role of our past in our present or our future work. I know I certainly had not until now even considered how far such discussions were relevant until the current pressing debate about where traditional acupuncture, previously occupying the centre of acupuncture's stage, must reposition itself or be forcibly repositioned by others in the universal health care system into which, often despite itself, it is now becoming absorbed. If they are to have any value in what they offer, all traditions must remain alive, and to remain alive all things, from a tree, to our bodies and our thoughts, must slough off any dead wood which may impede its growth, like a tree its dead bark or our bodies its dead cells. I am not sure that we do enough to distinguish the dead from the living cells of our acupuncture inheritance, nor even agree the necessity for doing this. And here I am as much at fault of taking at face value many of the traditions I have inherited as anybody else.

CHAPTER 7

MASTERY

People seem to throw the word 'master' around rather indiscriminately and, in my opinion, rather too freely. Why do I think this? To answer this I have had to ask myself what I understand by the word mastery. And even if we know what the word means, who is to determine to which person this should be applied? Many people can master a subject; that does not necessarily make them masters. In fact, often far from it. You can be hopeless at a subject, as I was in anything associated with mathematics at school, work hard to master it sufficiently to just scrape through an O-level, again as I did, but by no stretch of the imagination could other mathematicians call me a master of mathematics. It therefore isn't just a question of reaching a certain level in whatever area we are engaged in, but of something much more intangible than gaining a specific qualification or achieving a specific, presumably high standard. There is something else hidden in the word master which appears to raise the person to whom this word is applied to a more rarefied level, separating them off from what we can call the common herd, and placing them amongst the few. I like to think that it is an accolade, a mark of great respect, an acknowledgement of some special quality singling this person out.

I imagine that each of us may have a different under-standing of the word and bestow it on different people, depending on whom we have encountered in our life, so my definition here will be a very personal one, which may well not coincide with that of those reading this. To be added to the complex mix of how we have learnt to define mastery is a very personal factor. Have we been fortunate enough to come across a sufficient number of people with whom to make the kind of comparison necessary to gauge the relative skills of one person against another, for example? We must have the examples of enough people to assess one person's mastery and another person's inferior skill.

All this is no idle discussion, but has been prompted by something very personal, my own assessment that the person who taught me about five element acupuncture at the deepest level was JR Worsley, and my conviction that he merited the title of master. I know that I have therefore been privileged to encounter one master, and it is this encounter which has prompted these thoughts. The quality I recognised in him was something well beyond his having a deep understanding of his subject. It was something I learnt to recognise as a result of various en-counters I had with him over the years, some very personal to me and others witnessed by anyone privileged to be a student of his.

The first was a personal encounter, when I was in the role of patient taken by another practitioner to see him for a consultation. Before he came into the room I felt quite at ease, eager to see how I would respond to the great privilege of meeting him face to face. To my surprise, the moment he took my hand and asked me how I felt, I burst into a torrent of tears, almost as though his presence had unleashed the years of distress which lay well behind me and which I had thought I had dealt with. The interesting thing was that behind the tears was a feeling of relief and peace, as though the completely unexpected release of emotion had somehow cleansed me. I still remember thanking him through the tears and really meaning it.

So what had his mere presence done to heal me in this way? I thought a lot about it afterwards and in the many, many years since then, and my answer has always been that he had a capacity, through his eyes and his touch, to see and feel deep within me, a rare gift indeed. In the many years after this that I observed him with other patients, the same thoughts would strike me. He appeared to have the ability to understand another human being in a way I knew that nobody else could. That is what I call mastery, and I have always been proud to call him my master.

For me the word master therefore has a tinge of something intangible, something vouchsafed to only a few rare beings. Though each of us will experience a master's presence differently, for me JR Worsley's mastery was also encapsulated in what occurred one magical day in one of his classes in which he was to introduce us to more advanced point selection. He had his point reference chart in front of him, and went through the more than 350 points in turn, pronouncing the name of each almost as though chanting an incantation. It seemed as if he was re-acquainting himself with beloved friends. I could hear him murmur, 'Ah, this is a lovely point', or 'This point only a few people in the world are permitted to use', all elusive and tantalising comments to us sitting entranced listening to him. It was at this point that I became aware of the gulf between what he knew and was aware of, and what I would ever get to know. I knew then that he had access to another level of knowledge that I could never aspire to, however many years I practised. That is what I call the level of mastery.

If anybody calls me master now, as they often do in China, where the word is currently in much more common use than in the West, I always dispute this, and would like to reject the appellation. I am just thankful that I was once in the presence of an acupuncture master and had enough insight even in the early days of my practice to recognise this and take every opportunity to learn from his presence.

Do I wish I could call myself master? Not at all. It is enough for me to believe myself to be a good acupuncturist, and to strive each day to be a better acupuncturist. I know that my many years of study and practice have turned me into what others might even call a very good acupuncturist, but having been in the presence of mastery, I have been humble enough to worship at a master's feet whilst not seeking to emulate him or being concerned or even sad that this level has been denied me.

PART 2

IMMERSION IN THE ELEMENTS

CHAPTER 8

THE FIVE FINGERS OF A GIANT HAND

Occasionally we hear something that sets our thoughts moving in quite a new direction. One such instance occurred when I was listening to the radio some years ago, and heard the Astronomer Royal, Martin Rees, talking about the origins of the universe and making this startling statement: 'It could indeed be said that the universe was made for Man.' He had just pointed out that the chance of primitive matter floating down from outer space on to this tiny globe of ours, here to find conditions suitable for life gradually to emerge from the primaeval slime, was so infinitesimally small as to be discounted. Therefore, he continued, it would seem as if there had to be a purpose behind the creation of the universe which appeared to have us as its focus.

This is indeed a momentous thought, one which blew my mind when I first heard it, and continues to do so to this day. But what this also did was to add another dimension to my thinking about the world of the elements into which I move each time I enter my practice room. I have always marvelled at the ancient Chinese's ability to create universal concepts from simple, everyday terms taken from nature. Wood, fire, earth, metal and water all accompany us as natural phenomena throughout our life, from the warmth of the sun to the knife I use to cut my morning toast. There may apparently be nothing that appears to link these two concepts, the one which modern science has developed as defining the creation of the universe, and the other, the symbolic terms which the Chinese used to define all happenings including human life, and yet the elements, when viewed in all their fundamental significance, offer just as startling an interpretation of the origins of the universe as does that of modern astronomy. It is just that the language in which this interpretation is couched may appear to some to lack the scientific rigour expected of such discussions today.

When I heard Martin Rees saying what he did, I smiled to myself because the picture that it immediately evoked in me was that of a Michelangelo painting in the Sistine Chapel in which the hand of God stretches out to touch the fingers of Adam, our symbolic first ancestor, summoning him into life. This echoes the image of the five elements I always have before me, for I imagine them symbolically as together forming the five fingers of a giant hand, the hand of whatever God or creative principle in the universe we believe we owe life to. This giant hand hovers over all life, and, for some purpose of which we may only ever be dimly aware, it lays one finger on each of us as a blessing at our moment of conception, as though endowing us with some specific purpose associated with that one element's particular qualities, and thereby defining a direction which we are to follow and pointing us either East, West, North, South or to the centre, and thus to the element Wood, Metal, Water, Fire or Earth.

I cannot avoid thoughts like these when I write about what I do, although all those years back when I first encountered a five element acupuncturist at, of all things, a party in London I had no idea where this chance meeting would lead me. But like everything associated with my contacts with the elements since then, from my first treatment on, to my life as five element acupuncturist and teacher, and now, as here, to the thoughts that I have gathered together over the past years to fill my books, all has felt to me to be as though predestined, an inevitable progression. With my deepening understanding of the elements comes an appreciation of the profound philosophy which underpins all that I do. I remember JR Worsley telling us as students that there was always a part of every human being which belongs to the gods, and that with each treatment we must remember that we are being allowed by the patient to enter a sacred space. This made me aware that the calling I was now engaging upon was to do with the deepest areas of human existence.

Thus a study of the five elements, which can be regarded as the emissaries of whatever divine or other will created the universe, has become for me a fascinating examination of the purpose of human life, providing at the same time a highly effective discipline to treat the many ills, both physical and emotional, to which human beings can be subject. My understanding of the elements has therefore deepened with the years, as they have assumed profoundly different features from the rather basic, one-dimensional ones we were taught when I was a student. Then it seemed to be easy simply to see any expression of grief as inevitably pointing to the Metal element, or any expression of joy to Fire. It was only with experience that I began to see that these very simplistic generalisations rarely held true when I was faced with the complexities of a human being, for each of us is always a product of the combined qualities of all the elements. How to disentangle this great knotted skein of elements within one person to be able to trace one of its threads back to its source in a particular element was an often frustrating exercise in learning to be patient and give myself time, and has since developed into one of the most fascinating, though still often deeply frustrating, aspects of my work.

It delights me that what I have dedicated the past 35 years of my life to, and with luck and good health will continue to dedicate the last few years of my life to, has led me to explore areas of human life and our role in the universe in such a profound, infinitely surprising way. Every day I bless my fortune in having decided on that evening nearly 40 years ago somewhat reluctantly to don my party clothes and venture out into the cold of a December night to encounter, as I like to call it, my destiny.

CHAPTER 9

THE ELUSIVE GUARDIAN ELEMENT

In my writings I have made many attempts to capture in words the elusive qualities of the elements, and, within each element, the even more elusive qualities of the officials which do their work for them. Life never ceases to astonish me with its variety and unpredictability, and these are revealed in the different ways the elements offer themselves to our view. Just when I think I have a clear handle on one element, another of its qualities pops up unexpectedly to surprise me and to delight me, too. There is nothing more enjoyable than realising that the 'infinite variety' which Anthony saw in his Cleopatra is there in all of us.

The elements express themselves within us in many different ways. They have different ways of walking, of talking, of observing the world, of encouraging us in our choice of clothes, of deciding to do the work that we do and selecting the partners and friends that we do. The list is infinite, because it covers every tiniest aspect of the way we live our lives. Each element gives its own colouring to all the different choices we have to make at every minute of our life.

With time, of course, as practitioners of five element acupuncture we perceive in ever greater detail the different complex manifestations of each element, and become more awake to the little signals they send out containing all kinds of information about their states of balance or imbalance for the perceptive to note. It is these snippets of additional information that we add to whatever our senses can tell us, and in so doing put together an ever more complex picture of that person from which a dominant element will gradually emerge. I remember well the day when I was walking down the road and said of a young woman coming towards me, 'My goodness, she's got an absolutely white face; she must be Metal', and realising that I had at last developed sufficient skills to perceive her element from the degree of white on her face. Recently, too, I was startled enough to turn round and look back at a man whose path I had crossed, wanting to confirm for myself that he had indeed got a markedly greenish tinge to his face which led me to think how badly his Wood element must be out of balance. I am sure I would not have developed the necessary sensory skill to recognise either of these elemental colours a few years back. These are two instances of my increasing ability to translate sensory information coming to me in the shape of one element or another.

What I write about the elements is not intended just to help practitioners develop their practice. I hope it does that, of course, as does every study of the elements, but it does much more than that, because every time I write about the elements I am writing about life itself. And, as I have been told many times, readers of my books are not all practising acupuncturists but include lay people who are interested in discovering more about human nature. The elements are symbols for different physical aspects of the human being, such as our organs, but, at a much deeper level, symbols for life itself in all its variety. They are a way of understanding our differences as well as our similarities one from the other. The more we learn about them, therefore, the greater will become the depth of our understanding of ourselves, whether we use this understanding to deepen our practice, if we are acupuncturists, or just to grasp what is going on in people in general, if we are not.

The ancient Chinese symbols of the elements were first recorded in the earliest Chinese scripts more than 2000 years ago, but re-appear in Europe in mediaeval times in a different guise, that of the different humours which the medicine of the time recognised as describing human types. In a more modern context, too, they make their appearance in the work of psychotherapists, such as Carl Jung, where terms such as introvert or extrovert, passive or aggressive, imply a similar recognition of different human types. Jung, indeed, wrote that he wished he could see physical signs of the psychological types which he described. I would like to have been able to tell him that we as five element acupuncturists can and do see these, when we perceive the signatures of the elements in the sensory signals a person transmits through the colour of their skin, the sound of their voice, the smell on their body and their emotional orientation to life.

One way of looking at the elements is to think of them as stages along the path of any complete cycle, be it a life, a year or merely the development of a thought or the making of a decision, each of these stages having a quality all its own which distinguishes it from the other four. Thus all things relating to these five phases of life show similar aspects which differentiate them from those characteristics shown by the other phases. For some reason, of all the different species living on this earth, human beings appear to have been singled out as each having a particular affinity to one of these five elements, which forms the basis of our individuality. I do not think any other species has individual characteristics marked enough to differentiate them one from another in this way, although owners of some domestic animals, such as dogs and cats, or possibly also horses, claim that they have some of the individual characteristics we associate with humans.

I have called this element our guardian element. I like the name because it has overtones of the term guardian angel, and I think this is appropriate because this element assumes a strong protective role throughout our life. I think we are born under its protection, live our lives under its protection and die under its protection. Others maintain that it is not as constant a force in our lives as I think it is, but I have to leave it to my readers to make up their own minds. In my case, if I were to think that this element can change during our lifetime it would be a bit like saying that we can change our genes. We know that they do not change, and we know that the genetic imprint upon us marks us from birth to death and even beyond the tomb, when a sample of a dead body can yield as much information as that of us when we are alive. In the same way, therefore, I believe our elemental imprint is unchanging, and we can do nothing to alter it except to learn ways of developing its positive qualities to the full and minimising its negative ones.

This element appears to assume a dominant position within the circle of the elements, shaping each of our lives according to its characteristic qualities and with specific demands which it places upon us and which we need to fulfil if we are to live productive lives. We therefore live to a great extent under the control of this element, unable to shake off its influence. That this represents a truth is confirmed to me by each day of my practice, making it impossible for me to see things differently. Treating my choice of dominant element leads often to the kind of profound changes which treatment of any of the other elements does not. It is as though by reinforcing that specific element I have touched the very core of the patient.

CHAPTER 10

THE CYCLE OF THE ELEMENTS

I like to think of life as emerging gradually from the cosmos after the Big Bang, the moment at which the Dao, the All, split apart to form yin and yang and the five elements. Each element, in turn formed of its yin and yang duality, then assumes its own function of moving things forward, each creating individual stages through which life must pass on its way forward from birth to death.

To help us recognise the different signatures of the elements, we must first define in general terms the nature of the phases which together go to make up the complete cycle of activity represented by the elements. If we regard this cycle as forming an endless circle, we need to remind ourselves of the functions and qualities of the different elements as the cycle moves from element to element, each in turn created from its predecessor, as a child from its mother, fulfilling its function of moving the cycle onwards before handing over to its own child, the next element in the cycle.

Where then does such a circle begin and where end? It is customary to think of the Wood phase as its start, much as we may like to think of spring as the start of the annual cycle in nature, but if we examine this more closely it is also possible to consider things starting with Wood's precursor, the Water element, which nurtures the seeds from which Wood's buds will grow. Without Water's activities in winter there would be no spring. But then, without Metal's activities in autumn, life would not survive the winter months to enable those seeds to grow deep within the earth. And so on, back from element to element until we encounter Wood again, as each year circles round to produce another spring.

This is how we view the cycle of the elements in nature outside. If we continue this sequence on to the human level, we see this macrocosm reflected in the microcosm, in our bodies. Here the elements, differentiated into the various parts of the body, create our organs, and, at the deeper levels within us, our minds and our spirits. Each element therefore has control over specific aspects of our being. Occupied as we are with concentrating our attention at the level of the microcosm, which is the individual human being, it is good to keep this cosmic perspective in mind even when we are working at what may appear to be the more mundane, human level. I feel then that each treatment I give always remains tinged with a touch of the eternal.

I think it is important to think in this way because it provides a constant reminder of the awesome nature of what we do. We are not simply trying to cure a patient of a persistent headache. We are seeking to harness the power of the elements to help restore some disturbed balance between our patient suffering from a headache and the universal forces from which all life has sprung. If we concentrate all our attention only on the headache, we will achieve surprisingly little until we learn ways of embedding that headache within the widest context we can by relating it in some way to some malfunction of one or more of the elements. Then the elements themselves will respond in quite a different way, because we have tapped into the very depth of their connection to the Dao.

The five elements are phases of a complete cycle in whatever form this takes. They represent stages in the forwards movement which all things must be subject to if they are to move at all. Yin and yang, the first products of the Big Bang, alternate with each other and complement each other. They oscillate to and fro, but do not move from their position. If the world were composed only of these two alternating forces it would resemble somebody rocking back and forth from one foot to another, but never moving from the spot. The impetus which needs to be given to yin and yang to allow movement comes from the energy injected into the yin/yang duality by the differing actions of each of the five elements. Since each of them forms one stage in a complete cycle of movement, each adds a different impulse to the individual phases of this movement which represents the particular function which it is their task to perform. Nothing can be brought to completion until all five work together, just as nature cannot come full circle in a year without completing the cycle of the seasons. It is this cycle which propels the seed to become a bud, then on to full growth and fruition before finally stimulating the dying fruit to fall and be absorbed below ground to form the growth of new seed. Thus from Wood, bud, through the other elements to Water, seed, the five elements contribute what they are called upon to do, creating life, then eventually death and on to re-birth again.

As acupuncturists the aspect of the elements which concerns us most is how they manifest in each of us. As in nature outside, each of us is the creation of the elements, from the hair on our heads to the thoughts in our minds. I still find it awe-inspiring that the ancient Chinese were able to define the complexity of the human being so clearly in terms of the functions of these elements. It seems to me surprising that such a very profound understanding of both human anatomy and human psychology can have emerged in such a complete

form so far back in human history, some two and a
half thousand years ago, and probably even before that.
Every treatment I give offers proof of the accuracy of the
ancient Chinese understanding of the human being which
I cannot fault even after all these years. This is as true of
the psychological accuracy of what the elements tell us
about our emotional life as of the physiological accuracy
underlying their understanding of human pathology. This
understanding may be expressed in what may now seem
somewhat archaic language, and which some people may
not find befitting a modern form of medicine, but, when
applied to treating pathological conditions recognised by
Western medicine or psychological conditions recognised
by Western psychology, it proves remarkably effective these
several thousands of years later, indeed just as effective,
if not, in many cases, more effective than its Western
counterparts.

Much can be written about the differing characteristics
which each element imprints upon us. And this imprint
appears first as an expression of the different qualities
which each element imparts through the functions relating
to it which are the signatures upon the organs which they
create within us. Since each of us has a heart or a liver,
the qualities of that heart or liver are the products of the
elements, in the case of the heart that of the Fire element,
and in the case of the liver that of the Wood element.
In general terms, then, this imprint of an element upon
us will endow all of us with certain common features
characteristic of this element. We are all familiar with Fire's
sensory signatures, such as the colour red or the sound
of a laughing voice, and when the Fire element is strong
within us, we will reflect these sensory signatures strongly.
For example, we may laugh a lot, smell very scorched or
radiate great joy. Equally a weak Fire element will make all
of us less likely to laugh, or show little or no joy. All this

evidence of the strength or weakness of the Fire element within us will exert a common influence over us all, since it will just be a reflection of the work of Fire's organs, the Heart and the Small Intestine, which we all have.

To that extent there are common aspects to the characteristics which Fire imprints on us. But over and above these, there are other qualities which are under the overall control of the Fire element which contributes to defining a person's individuality. This is when the Fire element exercises the more dominant role of being the one element out of the five which it has been ordained (by whom, who is ever to know?) to take on the specific role of shaping our life much more individually, assuming the role of what I call the guardian element, and others call the element of the causative factor of disease (CF) or the constitutional element. At this more individual level, the characteristics of whichever element is our guardian element endow us with more specifically individual characteristics associated with that one particular element, colouring the whole sensory spectrum at a much deeper level, and giving increased emphasis to the outlines impressed upon us by this element. When the Fire element is strong whatever our guardian element, we will all show signs of happiness, but when Fire is our guardian element, the sense of joy it brings pervades every corner of our being in quite a different way from when we are joyful but our element is Metal or Earth.

In effect this particular element can, at a profound level, be seen as taking on the role of defining our destiny, of giving a specific shape to our life. Fundamentally this never changes, although we have some scope to fashion it in positive or negative ways. My element will always be Fire, but how far I choose in my life to develop Fire's qualities within me to the full, and therefore in a positive direction, or how far I restrict my choice and allow myself to pull my life out of balance and therefore in a negative direction, will determine whether I benefit or not from all that the Fire element can offer me. It is with respect to this aspect of our life that work can be done, both by ourselves and by those endeavouring to help us.

Of course the question of how much choice we all have to shape our lives is a great philosophical conundrum to which each of us has to supply our own answers. Like many others, I have wrestled with such questions, particularly since they have come to the fore in my work as acupuncturist. If each of us is endowed from birth with certain unique attributes created by the interplay of the elements, is there some purpose behind this, or is it merely a haphazard expression of the nature of things? I have come to believe that there must be some purpose, some direction for each of our lives, laid down for us at our birth. Others may disagree, and we are all free to come to our own conclusions on this. Mine have been increasingly shaped by what my practice has taught me, and in particular the understanding given me by my knowledge of how the elements dictate the way we live our lives, each uniquely according to how they interact one with another within us.

If a unique combination of elements controls my life and therefore how I respond to life's stresses, this shapes an individual destiny for me, defining how I respond to life's stresses. Since it appears to be our fate to live under the shadow of one element, we can, it seems, never free ourselves from its grasp, for we are determined by the specific qualities it endows us with from the day we are born until the day we die. We are unique manifestations of the interplay of the elements which together shape us, creating the organs of our body, the other physical structures in that body and the emotional structures which form our inner life, our spirit, our soul. If we accept that this is indeed so, this should have something to tell us about the need to consider whether this implies that there is a purpose to human life which is unique to each of us. If developed to the full, should we view this as an expression of an individual destiny?

This leads me to question how far we are each subject to the demands which the unique combination of elements forming us make upon us. Since these provide the structure within which we live our life, what freedom does each of us have to develop ourselves within this framework? What kind of a pattern do they shape us with? How far must we submit to the demands of this pattern, and can we indeed change it? If so, how far are we free to shape our own future, or is this future already decided for us?

As an acupuncturist using the elements as the tools of my trade, it therefore goes without saying (although it nonetheless needs saying) that my work with the elements therefore touches deeply upon the purpose of the individual lives my patients present me with, and certainly not just upon the mitigation of physical complaints. There is thus a depth to this work which I scarcely dreamed of when I started upon my acupuncture studies, though my own treatment had already given me strong intimations of this.

We can choose to ignore the implications of our obvious individuality, and thus not bother ourselves with trying to work out how far this should affect how each of us should live our life. Ant-like, we could prefer to remain as part of our human ant-heap from the time we are born to the time we die. And yet many of us, amongst these the most thoughtful, those with creative minds, wrestle with such thoughts throughout our lives, making them the main focus of our thinking. Is this not what Hamlet does, his 'to be or not to be' a profound examination of the purpose of life, perhaps the most famous expression of someone querying why we are here that there has ever been?

It is not then fanciful to think that each one of us potentially has an individual destiny, a personal challenge, like the one facing Hamlet, which we have been given as a task to fulfil during our lifetime. Here I note how often I wish to place the word 'potentially' in each sentence I write. For the gifts with which the elements endow us are merely potential gifts, things we can achieve only if we choose to. What then can turn the potential into the actual?

From where has come this conviction that my work at its deepest level is concerned with exploring such profound issues? The answer lies in the changes I observe in my patients after treatment. It is not simply that patients' physical symptoms improve, though that is certainly so in, to me still, a surprising number of cases. It is that I, and they, observe often startling changes in the whole direction of their lives. They appear different, sometimes almost unrecognisable from the person who first came through my clinic door, as though their treatment has caused a significant shift in the direction of their lives.

And where this impinges on five element acupuncture, which is what I am discussing here, is that this places upon its practitioners the task of determining, through their choice of element upon which to focus treatment, in which direction their patient's efforts at developing a meaningful life should lie, and then so strengthening this element that it learns to extend itself to the maximum of its abilities.

CHAPTER 11

SHAKING ELEMENTS OUT
OF THEIR COMFORT ZONE

We know that there is a particular emotion that is one of the characteristics of each element, there being five different emotions for the five elements. Together they cover the whole range of our emotional life, all contained within the five simple umbrella words of anger, joy, sympathy, grief and fear. Different acupuncture traditions have some variations on these descriptions. For example, Earth's sympathy is also described as 'thoughtfulness', although this is something I have never quite understood to be an emotion. But all are attempts to define in the most comprehensive way possible a fundamental emotional quality peculiar to that element.

I have always found it fascinating to receive confirmation daily from my practice and from my observation of human behaviour that these five emotional categories can indeed be extended to cover the whole gamut of human emotions, provided that it is understood that, like their respective elements within us, all are coloured by tinges of the other emotions, creating a human expression unique to each one of us. There is never just the emotion of anger in its pure form in a Wood person, because it will always include colourings of the other emotions which the elements within us add to the mix. To that extent, none of the sensory expressions of the elements can ever be considered a pure reflection of the description traditionally given it. The colour blue or the singing sound of voice will always contain within it shadings of other colours and sounds seeping into them from the other elements to be added to the Water element's blue colour or Earth's singing voice, and thus giving them that unique shade or timbre which characterise the unique human beings we all are.

Because of an element's close association with a particular emotion, people of that element develop a particular relationship to it, making them more at ease with this specific aspect of life because of its familiarity to them compared with the emotional areas controlled by the other emotions. As practitioners, then, we have to learn ways of familiarising ourselves with emotional approaches to life each of which may be slightly alien to us. I often like to quote the well-known saying by an 18th-century writer, Robert Owen: 'All the world is queer save thee and me, and even thou art a little queer.' However tolerant of other people we may claim to be, most of us are still critical when we encounter behaviour which is slightly at odds with ours. We may try hard for this not be so, but we will always tend to be disturbed by such differences. It is precisely this feeling of oddness which, if we are properly attuned to it, should point us in the direction of an element not our own. And then we must work out ways of learning to differentiate these other elements one from the other. If we pay attention to what it is about it that we find uncomfortable, this is often a useful signpost to another element. Rather than allowing ourselves to be disturbed by its unfamiliarity, we should welcome it for what it is teaching us about other elements. We will also find that, as we get used to tracing back all these pointers to different elements, our increasing understanding of the behaviour of elements gradually helps us build up an accurate repertoire so that we start to recognise more and more quickly the elements which are the trigger for this.

At different times we all display the whole range of emotions associated with the five elements. One way of helping ourselves become more alive to the differences between these emotions is therefore to think back to any situations which have led us to experience them ourselves. I am sure that we have all at different points in our lives felt ourselves in the grip of fear (Water), longed for some understanding of what we are going through (Earth), become irritated by somebody (Wood), wanted to share our happiness with others (Fire), or retreated into ourselves to deal with some loss (Metal). At different times we will express each of these emotions reflecting reactions to the different stresses each element is being subjected to, irrespective of what our dominant element is. We will therefore have at least some inkling of the effects within us of these different emotions. If we extend this understanding to what we feel a patient of a particular element may experience as their dominant emotion, this will go some way to feeling ourselves into elements which are not our own. It requires some persistent work to do this in such a way as to give us accurate feedback, but once we recognise how much our work is enhanced by an ability to understand within ourselves the emotional responses of patients of other elements, this will be an enormous help in pinpointing the right element and therefore responding appropriately to its needs. For each element demands responses which will reassure it that we recognise what these needs are.

It is not only that we all feel more at ease in the familiar company created by our element, and therefore tend to think other people will be as well, we also like to spread our particular emotional sphere around us by trying to draw other people into it on the assumption that this is what these other people want as much as we do. We therefore live our lives enveloped within a kind of a cocoon which our particular element spreads around us, and in which we inevitably seek to draw those who approach us, since this is the emotional atmosphere we are familiar with.

It is a useful experiment for us as five element acupuncturists to observe our own interactions with others very closely to see what kind of an emotional net we spread around those we meet. We may be surprised to note, as I was, how often what we are offering others in these interactions is not in fact what they want. In normal social situations this will not matter too much as we have all become used to accommodating ourselves to whatever the people around us demand of us, and usually manage to shrug off what we find irritating. In a clinical situation, however, things are very different. We are not there to demand of our patients that they cope with approaches which disturb them, but our task is to adapt ourselves through our knowledge of the elements to what will make our patients feel sufficiently comfortable to relax and be themselves. This is often the opposite of what happens in the world outside the practice room, and unfamiliar as this will initially be as we learn our craft, how successfully we manage to do this will depend upon some persistent work on our part.

So how do we go about learning the art of studying the emotional characteristics of each element? As usual, it is always good to start from what we know, which is our own particular element, and then gradually work outwards from that to each of the other emotional areas. We may think that we know enough about ourselves not to need to study our own element in great depth, but this is not so, and can be a form of self-delusion. I became aware of this when I started to observe myself more closely and found that I really had not until then realised fully how I appeared to other people and what effect I, and therefore my element, Fire, had upon those I encountered.

We take so much in life for granted, and perhaps we have to in any normal, social situation, otherwise we would spend too much time dissecting and analysing everything that is happening to us to get on with the actual task of just living. But as acupuncturists we have a different role to play. Here we need to be hypersensitive to all the little nuances which characterise our interactions with others.

So at times I have set myself to watching myself as closely as I could, observing my reactions to other people and theirs to me, and was surprised at how different some of these were from what I had assumed. By looking at what surprised me, I learnt a lot about how the Fire element, my element, is perceived by other people, and how, in turn, this element in me responds to the reactions of others. The main area of surprise for me was to notice how often the impetus for any approach to other people came from me. I would be the one to make the first move, often not giving others the chance to initiate the encounter even if they wished to. It was as though I leapt across the divide between me and another person as quickly as I could, because somehow the existence of the distance between us was slightly threatening.

So how does this behaviour of mine act itself out in the practice room? Again I observed myself carefully to see whether my instinctive rather rapid movement towards my patients was welcomed by them and therefore appropriate, or whether I felt something about it made any of my patients uncomfortable. What I realised was that my many years' experience must obviously have had their effect upon me, and altered my behaviour sufficiently to encourage me to rein in what is my natural exuberant welcome to anybody I meet, replacing it instead with approaches which differ, sometimes only slightly, but sometimes quite markedly from what I would consider natural to me. I saw that I must have learnt enough from my years of practice to adapt myself in different ways to what I could sense patients wanted from me. Such observations of my often instinctive adaptation of myself to the different elements my patients presented me with in turn added to my understanding of what each element felt comfortable with in the practice room. And here are some of my conclusions, drawn together for each element.

Fire, naturally, represents the approach with which I am most at ease, since both patient and I enjoy the same kind of emotional atmosphere around us. What I have to beware of, though, is not to allow myself to be lulled into relaxing too much and therefore overlooking subtle signs which may hint at problems which the patient is reluctant to draw attention to for fear of introducing a discordant note into what may perhaps be too cosy an atmosphere. I therefore have to be careful not to allow my own sense of relaxation at finding myself in the familiar environment of my own element make me perhaps unconsciously overlook what doesn't quite fit into this. It can be too easy just to relax, but I must never forget that I am not here to make myself feel comfortable, but to help the patient. This may require injecting a slightly more jarring note into what is going on in the practice room.

It is worth looking at why we need to do this. Presenting an element with a challenge of any kind reveals more about this element, and in particular about its state of balance or imbalance, than carrying on a treatment more in tune with what this element is comfortable with. Depriving an element of what it feels easy with forces it out of its comfort zone as it tries to adjust to what may be unfamiliar to it. Not to respond to the Fire element's smiles, for example, makes it sufficiently uneasy often for it to redouble its efforts as it attempts to coax something more from the person they are addressed to. By doing this in the practice room you are in effect not allowing the

Fire element to settle into its normal routine. By rattling things around a little you are therefore giving yourself the opportunity to observe how an element responds when it is jolted out of the kind of response it normally expects. Since we are trying to find out the kind of stresses which our patient experiences and which have prompted them to seek us out for treatment, we are creating for ourselves a situation which to some extent mirrors the real-life stresses they experience in the world outside.

But of course in all that we do we are also checking whether we are receiving confirmation that our diagnosis of the element concerned is the right one. By responding with slightly less warmth to a patient's warmth towards us may cause stress if their element is truly Fire, but receive an absolutely indifferent response from other elements, such as Wood or Metal, neither of which is looking to us for the closeness Fire enjoys.

So let us now see what Wood wants of me in the practice room, and how I will go about introducing a slightly disharmonious note into our interaction with people of this element which will tell me more, first about whether the patient is really Wood, and secondly how the patient copes with the slight stress this may cause them. I have always seen that what the Wood element wants above all can be summarised in the following two words: order and structure. Wood's function is to make sure that what it does, and those around it do, fits properly into a clear framework. Its task is to provide such a framework. What it expects from treatment is that the practitioner should provide a satisfactory, ordered framework for treatment. Because of this, Wood can be regarded as perhaps the easiest element into which to inject a slightly discordant note into the practice room.

Since the order with which Wood is comfortable includes that of having properly hung pictures on the walls it faces, a slight sense of disorder can be introduced merely by tilting a picture on the wall a little so that it hangs at a slight angle, and then waiting to see whether the patient notices this. I still remember with a smile one of my Wood patients lying on the couch in my practice room, surveying the ceiling above his head and informing me that the walls of my practice room were not aligned properly. He made it sound as though this was some kind of personal affront to him, and that it somehow offended his sense of what was appropriate in a practice room. All of this was confirmation indeed that his element was Wood.

I could not imagine a patient of another element, such as Earth or Water, being interested enough to note this, or, if noting it, as Metal or Fire might do, being concerned enough either to point it out to me, which might be Metal's reaction, or being reluctant to appear to be criticising their practitioner, in the case of Fire. Even in such an apparently insignificant episode like this, which involves merely turning a picture slightly on a wall, we can see how different the responses of the different elements can be, and how diagnostically significant these responses can be.

What about Earth then? What will shake it out of its particular comfort zone? And, for Earth, more than for any other element, it is a comfort zone which it wants above all. It searches for the safety of having its feet firmly grounded in whatever situation it finds itself in, and will not take lightly finding itself in situations which shake the ground beneath it. Although seeing a picture on the wall hanging at a crooked angle or having its practitioner laugh too much will not disturb it sufficiently to shake it out of its equilibrium, on the other hand not being allowed to tell you all it wants to in as much detail as it wants, and with as much repetition as it wants, will. Its principal function is, mentally, processing its thoughts, and, physically, processing the food it takes in. As practitioners we can't interfere with its physical function, but we can certainly interrupt its mental function, perhaps by not allowing it to finish a sentence it has begun, or not complete a story in as much detail as it wants. And Earth wants to include as much detail in whatever it is telling us so that it can be sure that we understand exactly what it is trying to tell us.

So to interrupt Earth's train of thought, hence its speech, is to deny it the possibility of spreading before us the detailed explanations and descriptions which it needs to get across to us if it wants to be sure that we understand what it is telling us. Earth people can indeed almost ignore any interruptions to their often quite lengthy exposition of some event that has happened to them, for fear that they will lose their train of thought. It therefore requires quite an abrupt change of direction with the practitioner interrupting the Earth patient's narrative to bring the patient to a halt. And even then, I have noticed with amusement that they will resume what they are telling me about as soon as I have ended my interruption at the exact point at which I interrupted them, often returning to the subject by saying something like, 'and as I was saying...'

An interruption to a Water person takes quite a different form and has quite a different aim. It is to startle, and hence to see whether this prompts the Water patient to show some of the fear always lurking below the surface. Just as it is easy to knock Wood off-kilter by hanging a picture on the wall slightly askew, so it is easy to startle Water simply by making some unexpected, abrupt movement, such as coming rather noisily into the room, or shutting the clinic door with a slight bang. Even saying with a startled sound in the voice something like, 'Oh dear', in reply to what the patient is telling us may prompt the patient to show some anxiety, as they wonder whether we think something is worse than they think it is.

Anything unexpected will rattle Water, so it is fairly easy to think of ways of startling it. It may show this through a physical movement, such as swivelling round to see what is causing the interruption, or, an even more representative pointer to Water, darting only its eyes whilst leaving the remainder of its body still, as a frightened animal may do when locked in the glare of a car's headlights. Water's eyes are unconscious mirrors of this fear; their rapid movements as they attempt to locate whatever is disturbing them, and often whilst trying to keep the rest of their body still, may often be the only indicator of hidden fear, whilst the rest of their body may appear to be relaxed, giving the illusion of indifference to what is going on around them. But Water is always immersed in a sense of suppressed anticipation and apprehension, ready to leap away either physically or emotionally at the first hint of danger. If we do something which Water may interpret as a potential risk to itself, we will immediately see by the speed of its reaction whether we are indeed dealing with a Water person. No other element will respond so quickly and so fearfully to any unexpected action of ours.

And so finally to Metal, perhaps the most difficult element physically to shake from its composure, but also perhaps the easiest to be affronted by some inappropriate behaviour on our part, and therefore to show its true colours. What Metal most appreciates is to be given respect, and in our dealings with it we have to show that we value it appropriately. How, then, do we act out some behaviour, for however short a time, which gives it the feeling that we are somehow undervaluing it, and in so doing give it a slight jolt to make it briefly lose its equilibrium?

I have been trying to think of past instances when I have felt that I have somehow miscalculated my approach to a Metal patient, and have been made aware of this by some reaction indicating, in however small a way, that the patient was not happy with something I had said or done. And I realised this has usually been as a result of some verbal misjudgement, in other words something I had said in a somewhat clumsy way, which has upset the patient. Thinking back on this, I realise that the factor common to these incidents has been over-hastiness on my part in suggesting to my Metal patient that they need to alter their behaviour. This can be seen as reinforcing an assumption that I somehow know what is best for the patient, or at least know better than the patient what they should do. In other words, I am implicitly judging that their opinions are less valuable than mine, thus reducing their sense of their own worth both in my eyes and theirs. And what matters most to Metal is to learn to evaluate its behaviour on some scale it has set for itself. To be forced to accept that another person knows better how it should conduct itself by allowing this other person, in this case me, its practitioner, to tell it how it should behave is to judge itself as in some way inadequate.

So how would I carry out an interaction of this kind as smoothly and as gently as possible so as not totally to lose a Metal person's trust, whilst at the same time ensuring that I press the right buttons to give it the kind of slight jolt which tells me that what I am doing has homed in correctly on the Metal element rather than on any other element? One way of doing this is to suggest that a way of behaving which the Metal element has decided upon may not be the best way by saying something like, 'I wonder whether it would be better if you...' Metal is unlikely to appreciate the slight criticism inherent in what I am suggesting, for the very reason that it implies that it has not done something quite right, an implicit rebuke, or at the very least a slight criticism. I cannot think that any other element would interpret this or be disturbed by this in such a way.

PART 3

Being a Reflective Practitioner

CHAPTER 12

WE ARE INSTRUMENTS OF NATURE

We were always being told by JR Worsley that we were to see ourselves as instruments of nature, a phrase I have always loved. It reminds me constantly of the connections which embed us, patients and practitioners alike, in the world around us. The elements with which I work, and whose signatures upon my patients I try to trace, form the lines of communication between the inner worlds of our souls deep within us, our bodies which house these souls and what lies outside these bodies of ours. Through our treatments we attempt to clear away as much rubbish as we can from the clutter of a patient's life to allow the elements in all their purity to fulfil the tasks they are called upon to assume. In some senses we could therefore regard ourselves as though in acting as instruments of nature we are also acting as instruments of a patient's individual destiny.

It is also good to ask ourselves what the purpose of what we do actually is. This is not something we often think about, regarding it as self-evident, but it is a question worth considering carefully when we look at the kind of help we wish to give our patients. We can give all the obvious answers, such as 'to treat physical problems', 'to make patients feel better'. But if we recognise that our treatment can heal a person by bringing harmony to them at the deepest level, what does such healing consist of? One of the things patients have often said about how they experience the effects of treatment has struck me as very

significant here. In different ways they have told me that
they feel 'more themselves', or 'know now who they are',
a recognition of some innate understanding we have of
something inside us confirming our own identity. When
asked, they have not been able to describe these feelings
in greater detail, but they know what 'being themselves'
is, even though they can't formulate it more precisely than
that. It always appears to be accompanied by a sense of
greater well-being, a feeling of something very familiar, of
returning to a long-lost but well-remembered place. 'Ah,'
patients seem to be saying, 'I recognise this place. I feel at
home here. This is where I feel truly who I am.' I might
not have regarded this as an effect of good treatment if
I had not had many examples of patients telling me just
that, and if I had not had my own experience to think
back on.

So who exactly is this person we each in different
ways recognise with relief as being a true representation
of who we really are? In my own case, I still remember
clearly the feeling of surprise which treatment brought
me that at a deep level within me I had discovered some
truth about myself and my connections to the world in
which I lived about which I had until then been unaware.
It was not simply that my treatment had made me feel
contented and at peace, which it did, but that there was a
familiarity to this feeling. Thinking back carefully to my
own experience, it represented a re-discovery of something
I had lost rather than the discovery of an entirely new
aspect of myself. I can find no other way of accounting for
the speed with which I accepted the changes I experienced
within myself, as though they were re-awakening a self-
evident truth about me. You could say that the 'I' whose
existence was confirmed in my saying to myself 'now I
know who I am' was an old acquaintance of mine, and

it would therefore be truer for me to have said to myself, 'now I know again who I am'.

Do the elements within us retain a memory of some pure state of being which represents who we are unencumbered by the distortions life has subjected them to? I think that it is possible that they do. This seems to be the only explanation I can offer to explain this sense of rediscovering our true selves as a result of treatment. Feelings like the ones I have described are only awakened if I address this dominant element out of the five. Patients may well feel their health improves if I concentrate my treatment on a different element, but not to this extent and not so quickly. I have found that it is only by addressing the right element among the five that such profound feelings of well-being are awakened, further confirmation to me, if confirmation were needed, that we do each have a dominant element, for this is the only element to respond in such an emphatic way when treatment addresses it so directly and so specifically.

It is by listening to the demands of this element that we appear to fulfil whatever destiny life has chosen for us, and it is by denying these very demands that we deny this destiny, and in so doing allow imbalances of both body and soul, and usually of both, to creep in.

CHAPTER 13

'Practitioner, Know Thyself'

The aim of any therapy can be said to be an attempt to effect some change in a patient's life, each therapy trying to do this in a different way – physical therapies through the patient's body, psychological therapies through the patient's mind and spirit. The interesting thing here, of course, is the almost unique fact that as five element acupuncturists we combine both roles, that of therapists treating both body and soul. We cannot ignore our own role in all this. Each therapist will bring themselves to the treatment and cannot avoid doing this. There is a two-way process here, in some therapies more acknowledged, maybe indeed more welcomed, than in others. In our training as five element acupuncturists we spend much time examining the subtleties of the patient–practitioner relationship, and the importance of shaping it appropriately to answer the patient's needs. That means, of course, that we have to be open to those needs and be aware of how far we ourselves as therapists may be unconsciously submerging our patient's needs beneath our own. I call this casting our own shadows over our patient.

'Physician, know thyself' is probably the most important lesson we must all learn if we are to presume to help one another. And the belief that we can help somebody else can indeed be regarded as somewhat presumptuous, unless we are sure that we are approaching our work with sufficient humility, and not with a hidden sense bordering on arrogance that we 'know' better than the patient what is good for them, what we might call having a hidden agenda of our own. It can be all too easy to allow an unconscious desire for power to enter into this relationship. Patients are after all often all too flatteringly grateful for our interest in them and we may allow this flattery to go a little to our heads. This is a natural human weakness which we must be aware of and resist.

And what does 'knowing ourselves' consist of? Above all it means being honest with ourselves, and examining our motives for doing what we do. Presumably we all enter a caring profession such as acupuncture with the aim of helping others, a noble-sounding yet vague aim which can, unless we are careful, hide a multitude of less noble motives. I asked each student who wanted to study at my college why they wanted to come, and all said that it was because they wanted to be of help to others. And then I would see some of them further on in their studies unable to cope with the realities of learning to deal with the demands their patients made upon them. It takes experience for a novice practitioner to stand back and observe their own reactions to their patients and to develop enough self-confidence to admit their own failings and work out ways to counter them. To 'know yourself' therefore implies that the knowledge of yourself that this gives you requires that you are humble enough to accept the need for changes in your own behaviour towards your patients, if you find that these are necessary. Each patient then becomes an exercise in self-development.

Not many people will be aware of this before they embark on an acupuncture or any other therapy course. I certainly was not all those years back, and only the experience of many years of practice has taught me this essential ingredient in the development towards becoming a competent and caring practitioner. For we always remain at heart the person we have always been, though, like cheese, we inevitably ripen with age. Whether at the same time as ageing we also mature depends upon the clarity of our insights into ourselves and, yes, yet again, the humility necessary to acknowledge our defects and the inner strength to try to correct them.

This, of course, applies to the whole of our life, not just to that small part of it which encompasses our work as a five element acupuncturist, but since this work involves the intimacies of a close relationship with our patients, it becomes all the more important that our own part in this relationship should be as balanced as possible, and that we should be as transparent to ourselves as to our motives and as to any personal agendas we have as is humanly possible. To achieve this is really a lifetime's work, as we learn to adapt to all the conflicting demands placed upon us at different stages of our life. But the important thing is that we recognise the need constantly to examine all aspects of our own development as practitioners so that we become aware of any personal problems developing in our relationship to a patient as soon as they start making themselves felt.

It is good for each of us to think what particular qualities we bring to our practice, because these will dictate the nature of our relationships with our patients. I like to use the five elements as a rough template for this, regarding each element as bringing a particular range of qualities to the practitioner whose guardian element it is. And just as we cannot escape our element's imprint upon us, we can no more escape its imprint upon our practice. This is something that is little discussed, perhaps because nobody has considered it a subject worthy of discussion. Having observed many, many practitioners over many years, I am convinced that a crucial element in the development of good relationships with our patients stems from a practitioner's own ability to understand the interactions which occur between them and their patients, taking their own element's orientation towards such relationships into account. Each of us, whatever our element, will, I hope, want the very best for our patients, but may find ourselves tailoring their wishes according to our own orientation to life, there being no such thing as neutrality in anything we do. This certainly does not matter if we accept it as a given, but one which we must constantly be aware of, since, if we ignore it, we may run the risk of interpreting our patients' needs according to our own perceptions, and thus misinterpreting them.

Life grants us many ways to help us understand both ourselves and other people, because, unless we live as hermits alone on a mountain-top, we live this life at all times surrounded by the many hundreds and thousands of those we encounter, each person providing us with a lesson on how to recognise the elements if we choose to do so. Nothing can equal the value we gain from being alive to each encounter we make with our fellow human beings wherever these are, whether in our family, at work, out on the street or simply sitting back and watching people on TV. All of these offer excellent opportunities for observing the elements in action, and provide a constant stream of examples of the different templates of the elements which we learn to draw together as our practice develops.

I enjoy watching how families or groups interact with one another, or how much eye contact a person I pass in the street makes with me, whether they are aware enough of others to step aside to let me pass or seem oblivious to the presence of other people. All these subtly different interactions can be used to teach us greater sensitivity, and help us take this heightened level of awareness with us into the practice room. No interaction with another human being is therefore a waste of time, and only becomes so if we do not make use of it to feed our practice.

This makes sitting in a café or in the park watching the world go by almost as valuable as observing one patient after another, and perhaps of even more value because the supply of fresh examples is potentially as limitless as the number of people who surround us. Though we get no direct feedback as to whether the element we think we are observing is the right one, the flow of so many different people passing before our eyes trains these eyes of ours and with luck, too, some of our other senses, to develop greater sensitivity.

But most importantly of all, we have to learn to watch ourselves, for therein lies the secret of how we learn to develop a deep understanding of the elements. Theoretically this should be the easiest thing of all for us to do, but in practice, human nature being what it is, it is not. For none of us is good at observing ourselves with as objective and clinical an eye as possible, so as to help us judge accurately our weaknesses and our strengths. We are all likely to be guilty of building up for ourselves some often flattering image which evens out some of our less admirable bumps, with perhaps as few blemishes and signs of inadequacy as we can. I suspect that we all aspire to have qualities which we would like to think of as admirable, coming under the headings of words like caring, unselfish and generous. We are less likely to want to acknowledge those other common and very human qualities of selfishness and intolerance.

The opposite failing, and one which is equally far from true, can be an exaggeration of our negative qualities of the 'I know I'm a failure' or 'I always do the wrong thing' kind. Somewhere in between lies the truth about most of us. We are sometimes selfish and sometimes unselfish, sometimes caring and sometimes extremely uncaring. The secret to gaining an accurate and truthful a picture of ourselves is to look at ourselves coolly and dispassionately over time, observing how we interact with other people, and how we react to what happens to us so that we begin to build up an understanding of our own strengths and frailties, and, as five element acupuncturists, relate these to the balance of the elements within us. This helps us become aware of how our own particular elements may be helping or hindering our practice. This will be based upon the extent to which learn not to allow our inadequacies to disturb our interactions with our patients. A clear assessment of how the elements within us shape our approach to others will deepen our understanding of the nature of the elements and at the same time prevent us as far as possible from casting any shadows from our own elements over our patients.

CHAPTER 14

THE MYSTERIOUS
REALM OF THE SOUL

Why does five element acupuncture place such emphasis
on healing the emotions? And why have I always felt that
there is a need to single this out as being one of its most
characteristic features? I think the answer lies in my belief
that we need to pay more attention to something often
ignored in modern medical practice to the detriment of
health, but which is usually so self-evident that the old
traditional texts hardly emphasise this. The increasing
secularisation of the approach to matters of health in most
modern societies has led to the demotion of the emotional
and the spiritual in favour of excessive emphasis on the
physical roots of all disease, and this has denigrated those
aspects of human life which cannot be evaluated in physical
terms. A discipline such as ours, therefore, which recognises
the human being as a complete whole, consisting of body
and soul, offers often refreshingly new insights into the
origins of ill health and ways of restoring health. I feel I
have a duty to emphasise this as I see the deeper levels of
human existence, our minds, spirits and emotions, as often
neglected in conventional medical practice, though not, of
course, in the wide range of practices which come under
the heading of psychotherapy, the therapies of the psyche.

Before discussing how exactly five element acupuncture
addresses these deeper areas of the human psyche, I find
I must first look in greater detail at what I understand by
the two terms, spirit and emotions. I must try to define

my understanding of each term and gauge exactly in what the distinction between them lies. Is our spiritual life the same as our emotional life? Does it cover exactly the same area of our existence? As I think of the word 'spiritual', something stirs in me which differs totally from when I address the word 'emotional'. With anything to which I attach the word spiritual I immediately feel as though I am entering a sphere of life lying beyond that of our day-to-day existence. What is emotional, on the other hand, seems to me to stay fixed in the everyday, a term with its feet firmly on the ground. The problem, also, is that the spiritual comes to us laden with much baggage, for however much we may try to discount this it always has about it a whiff of the religious, an unspoken or at times spoken belief in one or other religious system.

This is not how I regard this term, or how I wish it to be understood by others reading what I am writing. To me, the spiritual relates to the deepest level of human existence, that ephemeral, intangible, awesome and ultimately unknowable part which defies capture by simple, everyday speech, but lies there within us for all to experience when we listen to beautiful music, read a beautiful poem or experience deep feelings. The Germans have a lovely word for this, 'erhaben', that which is sublime, and describes what lifts us from our everyday life and points us towards the stars, making of any experience something greater, deeper than the sum of its parts. With what is emotional, on the other hand, I feel that I stay attached to my day-to-day life, although emotions, too, can have their spiritual aspects.

A further, often awkward distinction I make is between the words 'spirit' and 'soul', which I see that I often use interchangeably, writing the one here and the other there, without any clear understanding of why I feel one is more appropriate in a specific context than the other. Thinking about this now, I realise that much that I have written about the difference between what is emotional and what is spiritual is similar to my choice between these two words, spirit and soul. Things of the spirit, though definitely emerging from a deeper level of human experience than things on the surface of life, the physical, in my mind have to yield their place to something even deeper, the level of the soul. For me, talking about the soul is to touch on the most profound aspect within us. Though I may use both words on occasions with little desire to to emphasise their difference, yet I reach for the soul, not the spirit, when I wish to touch upon that part of us which belongs to the gods and for which words such as ineffable or sublime are appropriate.

It might therefore seem as if my writings place undue emphasis on this area of my practice, whilst in reality I only feel I need to do this because so many other branches of modern medicine signally fail to address causes of ill health which lie beyond the range of the physically measurable. In effect, all my work, both my writings and my teaching, are attempts to redress the imbalance which has been introduced somewhat artificially into modern medical practice, as the equipment it devises and continues to refine to an extraordinary level constrains it to pay ever greater attention to only those areas which this equipment is able to evaluate. If the sophistication of the measurements of minute parts of the human body, invisible to the human eye, such as the components of blood and cell tissue, can yield astonishingly detailed information that no previous generation could have imagined, this naturally leads to a tendency to concentrate more and more attention, and consequently of course more and money, on refining the instruments which provide this information, at the expense of paying attention to areas of human life which can be far less easily explored, but which have preoccupied philosophers of life over the millennia. Even though what lies deep within us, our soul and its stresses and delights, is far less easily quantifiable or measurable than the components of our blood, this does not make it less worthy of study. It could even be said that it increases the importance of our trying to understand what drives our inner being to do what it does, and how this may and does have a profound effect on the body which houses it.

We should not shy away from exploring the mysterious within each human being, for it is often these mysterious regions which hide the clues as to what may be causing physical imbalances.

CHAPTER 15

THE THREE LEVELS OF THE HUMAN BEING

I often ask myself why I think that acupuncture is so important a medical discipline. My answer is that I believe it brings together what the modern world has often so arbitrarily divided. There are many medical disciplines which concentrate on our physical aspects, such as Western medicine or physiotherapy. And there are others which have become increasingly dominant, particularly in the Western world, such as all the different forms of psychotherapy and counselling, where attention is paid predominantly to emotional issues. Then there are some, like specific forms of acupuncture, with five element acupuncture among these, which see the body as being a physical envelope, but one which shelters within it those other aspects of mind and spirit, regarded as the deeper levels within us. They regard a human being as an indissoluble whole, the physical being always linked to these deeper aspects. We can call this deeper level by different names, and it is often called the emotional level. Here I prefer the word spiritual to emotional, but I use this term to cover both.

The human being can be regarded as being formed of three levels, the outer casing, the body, its deep inner aspect, its spirit, and nestled between the two, the mind, the mental level, which I like to think as an intermediary between body and soul. When I was a student I remember that we were told that patients can be diagnosed as being out of balance at any of these three levels, the physical, the mental or the spiritual. This is a distinction which I have found increasingly difficult to make, and it appears to have dropped somewhat off the radar, perhaps for that very reason. The distinction between a physical or an emotional imbalance is fairly clear, that between a mental and an emotional imbalance less so. And then we have to take into account that a serious imbalance at one level will trigger imbalances at other levels, since a human being is a connected whole, so to keep these levels separate is to make a somewhat arbitrary distinction.

One way I have devised to help me understand what differentiates imbalances at the mental from the spiritual level is to think of the mind as acting in the role of interpreter, with the task of interpreting the signals the spirit deep within us sends out. You can see this act of interpretation in the mental mechanics the brain has to perform in order to put our feelings into words. I can feel something at a deep emotional level, some reaction to listening to beautiful music or watching a lovely sunset, but the act of transcribing this feeling into a form which will enable me to convey what I am experiencing to another person through the medium of words requires input from another aspect of myself, this time my mind. The spirit has to ask the mind for help in formulating the words to describe what the spirit is experiencing. Similarly, the body has to ask the mind to fulfil a similar task in conveying what it is experiencing to what lies deep within us.

In the past, I have used a simple example to illustrate the interconnections between these three levels. If somebody has an accident in which they break a leg, initially this can be called a purely physical cause of an imbalance. If however, this broken leg prevents them from walking or driving the car, they then have to worry about how they are going to get to work or how they will get their children to school each day. Now their mind becomes involved and is placed under stress. Finally, if they cannot sort out the problems their broken leg is causing them both at home and at work, the worry is driven further inside until they become distressed and anxious and unable to function properly. Now all three levels, that of the physical, the mental and the spiritual, are under stress. Merely waiting for the broken leg to repair itself at a physical level will not help them if in the meantime they have lost their job or the leg may not be healing properly, putting yet more strain on the whole of their being. If you add to it any pre-existing areas of stress, such as those relating to family or work, the situation at all levels can become even more complex.

I often come across things people have said which express in different ways what I am thinking about at the time. When other people's thoughts resonate with me, they can add another dimension to my thinking, giving it greater depth. Here, then, is an example of another such thought relating to how I understand the deepest level within us. In an article in the *Guardian* newspaper about the importance of fostering creativity in schools I read the following: a headteacher from Hong Kong was said to encourage his students to sing together and play classical music. 'There's something', he said, 'that words can't describe, something deep inside. Once you tap into that thing, it gives life to everything else.' I can think of no better way to describe the difference between the mental level, which can use words to describe, and the spiritual level 'that words can't describe'.

At different times, different societies place greater or lesser stress on the different levels within us. A society in which religion plays an important role will be much more open to accepting those things 'which words can't describe' than a more secular society in which religion of any kind

plays an increasingly minor role. I can use an example from
my own life to illustrate the pervasive influence a religious
upbringing can exercise even on a younger generation
not subject to any strict religious practice. Although I
was brought up in a secular, half-Jewish family, with no
affiliation whatsoever to either Christianity or Judaism,
the stamp of my father's originally Christian upbringing
made itself felt quite clearly in the way he viewed Sundays,
the Christian holy day. My English grandmother went
to church each Sunday, and looking back I realise she
must have been shocked that her son did not follow in
her footsteps, although I never recall her ever making
this obvious to us, her grandchildren. But secular as our
Sundays were, my father still viewed the day as being
different from the other six days of the week, and in a
slightly quirky nod to his own Christian upbringing was
shocked if his daughters wore slacks on what he obviously
still thought of as a religious day, which demanded more
formal dress. This sense of Sunday being a day which was
slightly set apart has left a slight trace in me, too, in the
idea that somehow I should try to get my shopping done
on a Saturday, as though I hesitate to sully a holy day with
such mundane business. Wearing only skirts on a Sunday
soon disappeared without trace as I reached university, but
it must have left this slight memory behind, or I would
not be thinking of it now.

Why I am mulling this over at the moment is because
visits to China have made me aware that I enter there into
a culture which, despite many years as a predominantly
secular society under Communist rule, still attaches
greater importance to the spiritual side of life than is
generally the case in this country and perhaps in the West
in general. Of course, Sundays and festivals such as Easter
are not celebrated in any particular way as they are in the
West, except by the surprisingly large number of Christian

Chinese, but underlying everything is a strong respect for the deeper aspects of life. We can see evidence of this in their veneration of their ancestors and the respect they pay the elder members of the family. In the small area of life which I come into contact with as an acupuncturist, participants at my seminars have an instinctive understanding of the spiritual aspects of the practice of five element acupuncture which initially surprised me. I am always almost humbled, too, as I hear the students chanting in unison passages from the revered traditional medicine texts at the start of each day, much as though Western medical students were to recite passages of the Hippocratic oath before going out onto the wards. This chanting imbues the day with greater significance, even for me, the students' tutor, waiting in the wings to start the day's teaching.

That a deeper tone is set for all seminar participants in this way means that I experience teaching Chinese students as being in some way different from teaching their Western counterparts. In this country, by contrast, I have watched, increasingly sadly, as the training of acupuncturists becomes ever more mentally based. It is the mind which is set to work preparing research portfolios or MA theses. And in this work the spirit can become buried under torrents of words and ideas pouring into students' computers from all corners of the earth. There is then a danger that contact is lost with that deeper aspect of their patients, their spirit, which often cries out for attention.

In this context nature is a symbol for the fundamental principles underlying five element acupuncture, those represented by the elements. For historical reasons the Chinese have for many years encouraged their traditional medicine practitioners to develop their skills as though in tandem with Western medicine, and adhering to many of its principles. In so doing they have risked losing sight of the importance to health of the deeper levels of life.

In much modern Chinese acupuncture, indeed, the deeper levels of mind and spirit are to a great extent ignored, with emphasis predominantly on attempting to alleviate physical symptoms. Despite this, their traditional medicine practitioners have retained an innate understanding of these deeper levels, and have therefore found it very easy to integrate into their practice the kind of approach which five element acupuncture offers. My experience from my time in China in the past six years has shown me that Chinese acupuncturists have from the start a much quicker understanding of what I am trying to teach than that shown by most Western students. This shows itself in a surprisingly ready understanding of the importance of incorporating into what they do that often-ignored ingredient of life, its spiritual component.

I give below another lovely quotation which illuminates what I am writing about. I blogged about this some time ago, but it caught my eye again, in a slightly different context. I think it fits neatly into what I am describing here. It is an Indian proverb quoted by Rumer Godden in the preface to her autobiography, *A House with Four Rooms*.[1] Her writings all have about them a touch of the spiritual, as is emphasised here:

> Everyone is a house with four rooms, a physical, a mental, an emotional and a spiritual. Most of us tend to live in one room most of the time but unless we go into every room every day, even if only to keep it aired, we are not a complete person.

I like to think that my five element practice enables me to do just that: to spend rewarding time each day in these four rooms. For if a five element acupuncture practice remains only in the physical room we will become the incomplete practitioner Rumer Godden warns against.

---

1   Godden, R. (1989) *A House with Four Rooms.* London: Macmillan.

CHAPTER 16

GETTING TO KNOW OUR PATIENTS

If we are going to be of any help at all to another human being, as we as acupuncturists surely hope to be, then we have to make every effort to get to know the person who is coming to us for help. And getting to know somebody is certainly not as easy as it may sound, for each of us can present different faces to the world, having learnt during our life to adapt ourselves to the different people we encounter. The practice room represents an unknown world, and at first patients will be unsure both about the treatment being offered and the person offering this treatment. Practitioners, too, meeting an unfamiliar person, will have their own concerns to face in adapting to what is to them also a new situation.

All this represents different kinds of challenges. Patients are being asked to reveal something of themselves to a stranger about whose capacity for empathy and ability to put them at their ease they are initially unsure of. They will be asking themselves whether the practitioner is a safe person to whom to show any vulnerabilities, those which all of us may wish to hide from others, but which reveal the true nature of why we are seeking help. The practitioner, too, will be trying to adapt to the many different ways patients present themselves in the unfamiliar situation they find themselves in.

There is a great skill in helping a patient overcome their natural reticence at opening themselves up to another person. We have to learn ways of convincing our patients that we are a safe repository for self-exposure of this kind, and we need to know what kind of a relationship with their practitioner our patients feel comfortable with, since for each person this differs. Some, with a trust in human nature, will assume that anybody in the guise of practitioner will be worthy of this trust. Others, at the other end of the spectrum, will take much longer and request much greater evidence from their practitioner that the practice room is a safe place before lowering their defences.

The initial encounters between patient and practitioner are therefore delicate affairs, requiring great sensitivity on the practitioner's part to all the little signs we give out indicating where others must tread warily when they approach us. If practitioners do not pick up such signals, we are very likely to act too clumsily and thus effectively silence our patient. Here, as with all things, a knowledge of the elements comes to the practitioner's aid. For each element demands a different approach from us. And as we get better and better at analysing the complex nature of each approach, so this will give us increased insight into what may well be our patient's element.

The first step is to feel our way to the kind of atmosphere in the practice room that our patient appears to feel comfortable with. A good atmosphere is created when we feel our patients are responding easily to our questions with no hint of discomfort. But it is not simply a matter of appearing to look interested in what our patient is telling us or generally being sympathetic to the troubles they tell us about. This is the way we may react in the outside world when we hear the problems of people we are not very close to and say, with little real feeling behind the words, things like 'Oh dear, how dreadful', and then immediately move on to talk of something else. Society is very adept at laying this kind of gloss over any deeper emotional response. It is a way of satisfying the social need for people to show concern for others, but with no real intention to probe below the surface to find out what is really of concern. Most of our interactions with others tend to be at this level. After all we cannot become too involved with the troubles of too many people, for this may draw us into developing deeper relationships with them than we can ill afford to have or have little time for.

Therapists of any kind, though, have to enter into a totally different relationship with their patients. They are not asked to remain carefully on the surface of a patient's life, as those we encounter in normal social interactions are. They must probe more deeply to reach beneath the social veneer we all put in place, and set up a completely different kind of relationship with their patients, acknowledging that the practice room allows for, indeed demands, other approaches. And this always takes time. We should not feel that we need to be in any hurry. Patient and practitioner should gently ease themselves into a relationship which both find comfortable, and which allows the patient to feel the security needed truly to be themselves, to be the person they really are, which is not necessarily, and indeed rarely is, the person wearing the mask a particular society demands of them.

I was recently at a social gathering where those present each showed themselves with just such a mask on, something I was aware of because I have been thinking a lot about this recently. So I set myself to watch carefully what was going on around me, more carefully perhaps than I would usually do. And this careful attention paid off for me in the realisation that all these people I knew well, friends and relatives of each other, were skimming along on the surface of life in their remarks and their interactions to each other. I became suddenly aware of this when I, who have always been the kind of person who barges in where angels fear to tread, as the saying goes, started to say something very serious about the background relationships some of the group had with a particular person. Immediately I could feel the atmosphere change. One person in the group moved away, as if he hadn't been listening to what I said, and another quietly turned the talk in another direction.

I realised that I had opened up a brief glimpse into deeper, and therefore possibly darker and more complex emotional waters which obviously represented a somewhat disturbing area of life not suited to a purely social gathering like this. At first this disappointed me, but then I realised that I should not have interrupted what was a pleasant social occasion with what I should have known would be disturbing insights into deeper relationships within the group which only I was prepared to explore in this gathering. You could say that it was actually tactless of me to bring a totally different emotional atmosphere into what was simply a pleasant social occasion, and afterwards I was cross at myself for doing this. I suppose I am so used to what is demanded of me in emotional terms in my role as practitioner that I brought this role inappropriately with me into a social occasion where it certainly jarred.

But this has made me think very deeply about the very real difference between a patient–practitioner relationship and any other purely social relationship, reaffirming to me how very different these relationships are. And perhaps never the twain should meet!

CHAPTER 17

ALLOWING OUR FEELINGS TO GUIDE US

If we are to approach a patient's visit in the right spirit, we have to do some preparatory work in ourselves before the patient arrives. It is no good just expecting our senses and everything else that we have observed in our patient before to click into place as the patient comes through the door again. We need to think through what we have so far learnt about the patient and from the patient, and put this into some context in relation to whatever element we are proposing to treat. We must try to align ourselves with this element, using all those little pointers to its presence we have amassed from treating other patients on this element. This concentration within ourselves of all this then adds a proper focus to the impressions we receive as our patient comes into the practice room. These will often be fresh impressions because the patient may well have changed a little as a result of the passage of time and also, we hope, as a result of the effects of the last treatment. We will have built up a picture in our minds of how we expect them to present themselves, and this expectation may or may not be confirmed by how they actually appear before us. Maybe something we were expecting isn't there or something jars, somehow doesn't quite tally with how we assume the patient will be.

This is one of the questions we should always be asking of ourselves at each treatment. Does how the patient presents themselves fit with what we know of the element we have chosen, or does something not quite fit? The best time to try to find an answer to this is often our first impression at the next treatment. As a very salutary lesson which has stood me in good stead ever since, I remember well the moment when a patient I had treated for a long time on Earth (successfully both she and I felt) came to see me after a long break, and I suddenly realised that her colour was not the yellow I was expecting, but green. And when I followed this impression up by observing her carefully throughout the treatment, which I changed immediately to Wood, I could see all the little pointers to Wood, in addition to her colour, which I must have been overlooking before. She had a clipped voice, abrupt movements, and a take it or leave it approach to life not at all fitting the Earth picture I had thought was there.

Why had I not seen this before, I thought? Probably, I answered myself, because I had fallen back into the bad habit we can all have of assuming our diagnosis to be correct, and therefore feeling that we need enquire no further. In other words, I shut my patient up in a box I must have marked as Earth, and turned away from any closer examination. This was a big lesson to me never to take anything about my diagnosis for granted, but query it again and again, particularly if there has been a gap between treatment, and we are able to see our patient with fresher eyes.

The more experienced we become, the more we begin to rely increasingly on the feeling a person evokes in us. It is difficult to define what this actually means, but we all spend much of our lives relying on such feelings to direct what we do in relation to other people. This also holds true of our relations with our patients. We are taught in acupuncture college to recognise the elements through sensory signatures (sound of voice, colour, etc.), and although pinpointing these accurately is a very hard skill to learn, it is probably even harder to trace a feeling about a person that will help us identify the element which is stoking that feeling in us. As much as we need to practise by looking at many different people to determine their elemental colour or listening to their different voices to determine their elemental tone, we also need to practise the rather more ephemeral, less tangible skill of analysing the feelings people stir in us, and then learning to trace their origin to one element or another.

I had a good example of the need for this recently, one that echoes others I have had many times before, and which pointed me away from the element I had originally chosen to another element. I had diagnosed a patient as being of the Fire element, and would have happily continued treatment on this element except for a thought which passed through my mind the next day and which would not leave me alone. I found myself saying to myself, 'She's a very passive person, isn't she?' followed by, 'Could I ever describe Fire as passive?' I then thought of as many Fire people as I could, patients and friends alike, and realised that to none could the word 'passive' be applied.

This was a new thought to me, and added something to my understanding of Fire's natural energy. It is, after all, the element associated with the most yang, outgoing, time of year, high summer, a season which is brimful of energy, bursting forth wherever we look. Even when the person is a quiet kind of Fire, I still picture it as if it is always leaning forward actively to engage with others. So if I didn't think that this feeling of activity was typical of my patient, which element might it then be typical of? And I turned instinctively to Earth, because I could also picture myself in the practice room leaning over the couch as if to enclose my patient in my arms, realising that what I was doing reflected the feeling this patient gave me of demanding something of me. Unlike Fire, which always tries to offer something to others, she wanted me to offer something to her and I was responding to this need. This made me decide to change the element to Earth the next time I saw her.

Why had I not seen this before? That is, of course, the $64,000 question. We often see something which may be there, but may only be part of the picture, not the whole picture. I thought she had a pinkish colour and that she smiled a lot. In fact when I looked more closely, with the thought of the Earth element prompting me, I realised that this pink overlaid a wider spread of yellow over the whole body, and her smile did not warm me and light the room up as Fire's tries to do.

If we feel that something jars in us when we think of the patient, we must never let things rest, but make every effort to try and work out what is prompting this feeling in us. Sometimes, I have found, it can be traced back to something in the patient which reminds me of another patient, something perhaps as apparently insignificant as the way they look at me, or some specific way of talking. We must never ignore this, because this is usually nature's way of telling us something new about the patient which is likely to help us determine the underlying element. I sometimes have to wrack my brains to try to remember which of my patients this current patient reminds me of. If I can remember this it becomes a very helpful shortcut to the element.

I said that I had noticed that the skin colour of the patient I changed from Earth to Wood was overall a yellow colour. As part of our training as acupuncturists we were told that a patient's elemental colour could be seen at the side of the face, a colour glimpsed almost in a kind of a flash, and therefore like a passing shadow. I have always found this difficult to see and wondered at one point whether I was looking in the wrong place on a patient's face, until I realised one day after a few years of practice that I had discovered for myself a different way of detecting colour. It started with an experiment I did, when I asked students to stand next to each other in small groups, with the rest of the class looking at each person in turn as they changed positions with each other. What was surprising to me was the way the colours on each person's face appeared to change often in a quite startling manner when they stood next to people of different elements. This was when I first understood what Water's colour could be, often a transparent kind of blue, which changes quite abruptly when next to another element's colour.

This confirmed for me that there is definitely an overall colour on the face which differs from person to person, and not merely a shading on part of it. It also made me wonder whether the whole body skin reflects this element just as much as the face. By placing my hand against different parts of the patient's body, and watching to see how the colour I am seeing reacts with the colour of my own hand I have now learnt to see skin colour over the whole of the body as part of an element's signature. It always intrigues me now to see that when I place my hand against a patient's skin, it will immediately deepen to a stronger red tone (my Fire colour) when contrasted with the skin of a patient of another element, and will fade back to its more normal pinkish colour when laid against the skin of another Fire person. I can clearly differentiate the colour of a Metal person, for example, who in my eyes appears as though sheathed in a veil of white, from that of Earth with a warm, glowing yellow flush upon it. Because it is simple to compare my hand colour when laid against a patient's body skin, here then is one more practical and sometimes quite easy way of helping me see differences between the elements, thus helping with my diagnosis.

I am sure that all practitioners will find their own individual ways of identifying the specific colours, smells, sounds and emotions of the different elements, much as I have done. Using the information gained from previous patients we have treated we then learn to apply what we have learned to patients we are meeting for the first time.

I like to think of approaching each treatment as though asking a question, along the lines of 'Is what I see in my patient today consistent with what I have previously learnt about the element I have chosen to treat?' If the answer is 'yes', I continue treating that element. A negative answer requires that I must be honest with myself and accept that I have more work to do.

CHAPTER 18

Taking Our Time

The knowledge that deep within each of us there is a strong link to one of the elements which defines us and gives a direction to our life transforms what could be considered the burden upon us as five element acupuncturists of 'finding the right element' into what I regard as a blessing, a gift. It changes the calling I have chosen, or, I often feel, has been chosen for me, from simply being my day-to-day work into something akin to a privilege. My understanding of the elements gives me a precious tool, an elemental compass, which enables me to help patients adjust the direction of their lives and regain the path their element lays down for them.

How is it that treatment can make such adjustments possible? In deciding which element to treat we are in effect saying that we have chosen this one element out of the five as showing by its presence that it plays the most important role in this patient's life. We know it lays discernible sensory signatures upon us (colour, sound of voice, etc.), but there are many other ways in which it reveals its presence, and each practitioner's experience will have supplemented what our senses can tell us. And as I have said many times, it takes more years to develop these senses than most of us will admit to. It seems that nobody likes to feel themselves to be a novice here, particularly after some time in practice; it is only human nature for us to assume that learning to observe such sensory signs cannot be as difficult, as, after all these years in practice, I have learnt that it is.

It is therefore far better for us not to start relying simply on our senses at any stage of our practice, for sensory signs can be illusory, particularly if a more experienced acupuncturist is not around to give us feedback. Now that I know how long it took me to differentiate the rather hysterical laugh of Water under stress from the more pleasant Fire laugh, or the singsong Earth voice from the falling tone of a Metal voice, I realise that I was arrogant enough in the early days to think my diagnoses were accurate when they were not. Surely, we may tend to ask ourselves, it cannot be that difficult to identify a certain tone of voice or a specific emotion, can it? We all know what joy is, don't we? Yes, we do, but what only experience can teach us is that joy comes in many shades, and can be coloured by anger or grief, or hide fear. It is these subtle shades that experience gradually teaches us to detect, and experience only comes with time, and, crucially, with time plus humility. I have often heard with some dismay students and even practitioners declaring firmly that this patient is 'definitely Fire', or 'clearly has a shouting voice', their firmness, I feel, more to convince themselves than because they really feel they know. I am much happier if I hear somebody say, 'I think this is Wood, but I'm not sure yet', because, however experienced we are, we should all clearly regard ourselves as 'not yet sure' until we have enough evidence that that elemental compass I was talking about was leading us in the right direction, in other words, into the particular domain of one of the elements, this patient's guardian element. And this confirmation can really only be given by evidence from the results of treatment.

So once we acknowledge that pinpointing the sensory signs with accuracy takes time, there are, though, many other leads to the elements we can acquire to supplement what our senses tell us. The most important quality of all that we need to nurture within ourselves to help us here is that of training ourselves to be observant at all times, constantly on the alert to recognise signs of the elements in all the people surrounding us. That does not, of course, mean only our patients or ourselves, it means everybody we come into contact with. I am still surprised, though, when I see how little time students, let alone practitioners, spend in trying to trace the signatures of the elements in themselves, potentially the greatest source of learning if we are honest with ourselves. 'Practitioner, know thyself' is surely one of the most important lessons for all of us to learn who are in callings which claim to be there to help others, and it is important that we apply the lessons we have learnt from self-observation to our work with others. In doing so, though, we must remember that it takes courage to confront ourselves honestly and to learn to admit our own inadequacies, whilst, of course, to praise ourselves where praise is due.

We ourselves can prove to be the best learning tool for our role as five element acupuncturists, particularly in respect to our own guardian element, but also when attempting to learn more about all the other elements, since we can trace them all within ourselves. It is good then for all of us to observe ourselves when we find ourselves angry or frightened, sad, joyful or in need of comfort, experiences we will have in common with all humanity. And these personal experiences will teach us so much about how people of other elements live their lives. It is only by somehow getting into the skin of others, or rather below their skin, into the deepest parts of them, that we can really begin to understand what it is like for a life to be lived under the control of elements other than our own. And, if we are not self-observant, even our own element may remain a surprisingly unknown quantity to us.

We need to use all the signals the elements in our patients are giving us, because each in their different way tells us something, just as a word here and a word there will together go to make up a full sentence. Thus does a hint here and a hint there indicating one element or another eventually help us piece together a complete picture of an element. We must therefore never ignore the tiniest pointer to an element, because sometimes this is all we have at first to go on, and we cannot wait too long for this bigger picture to appear, since we are expected to start treating our patient at the earliest opportunity.

The first treatment will usually be given at our second encounter with our patient, after we have spent the first making a preliminary diagnosis. I have often thought that it would take some of the stress involved in trying to diagnose a guardian element if we could only give ourselves more time simply to get to know our patient. It is assumed that a psychotherapist, after all, will take many months, if not years, to learn how to help their patient. Why then the hurry with us, since we also include psychotherapy, the treatment of the soul, in our treatment? If we slowed everything down and allowed ourselves more time to engage with our patients, we would at the same time also be allowing the elements to reveal themselves more clearly, and thus make the process of pinpointing the dominant element quicker. I have, though, not seen anybody advocating this, nor have I so far done this either, because patients are, after all, coming for acupuncture treatment, which they expect to be about being needled, and not just to talk their problems over with their acupuncturist as they expect to do with a psychotherapist. I think, however, that we could adapt what we do much more in the direction of giving ourselves more time to get to know our patients in the round, rather than too hurriedly trying to concentrate on tracking down their element.

Taking more time before the actual treatments start would, of course, place a greater strain upon a practitioner's skill in establishing that all-important close relationship with their patients without which no treatment can be successful, however correct may be the assessment of which element to focus upon. The elements will often hide behind the social masks we all put up when we meet another person, particularly in the often difficult and almost threatening situation of a first encounter with a therapist. I often feel that not enough emphasis is given to this area of our practice in acupuncture training programmes so that novice practitioners are not made as fully aware as they should be of the overriding importance of this aspect. Redressing the imbalance by shifting the emphasis given to this by reducing the speed with which acupuncture treatment with the needles starts would help, but I see little chance of this happening or of others agreeing with my belief in why this is so important.

Be that as it may, we as practitioners can ensure that we give ourselves enough time to get to know our patients by including with each treatment a kind of continuation of the time taken over the initial diagnosis at our first meeting with them. A treatment, if effective, will change the patient a little, and sometimes a great deal, so that the person coming into the practice room next time is no longer the same as the one who came last time. We therefore need to find time at the start of each visit to widen our diagnosis to include what we have learnt from the changes which have occurred in our patient since we last saw them. Even if the treatment has not been effective, and there has been no change, this will also tell us something, revealing perhaps that the patient is disappointed or unhappy in some way, and here the manner of the disappointment or unhappiness will also tell us much about the patient's element, and needs to be explored further.

The time given to selecting which points to use and actually doing the physical treatment then becomes by far the shortest in the whole treatment, whilst the time taken

at the start of treatment to assess change or no change
and to conclude the treatment by observing whether there
are any fresh changes observed by us as the patient leaves
should together take up the major part of treatment. After
all, locating points and needling them does not take long,
even in new practitioners' hands. It is choosing the points
to correspond to what we have assessed as our patient's
needs on that day which takes the most time.

CHAPTER 19

TAILORING TREATMENT TO A PATIENT'S NEEDS

Perhaps one of the most important aspects in developing good treatment protocols is to assess carefully what kind of treatment we need to select to respond to a particular patient's needs. We were always told that what a patient needs is very different from what a patient apparently wants from treatment. Patients know what they want treatment to help them with, for these are the reasons behind their decision to come to see us. They are aware that something is not right and hope that the practitioner can help them put this right. They have no way of knowing what treatment is needed to do this, and must rely on the practitioner's competence to assess the situation accurately and select the right treatment. Patients and practitioners therefore see things from different angles.

Assessment of a patient's needs is really another way of describing the process involved in diagnosis. The problem with the word diagnosis is that it has a finality about it which is totally at odds with the progress of five element treatment. The word may be appropriate in the context of Western medicine, where certain diagnostic indicators, often carried out by some form of laboratory test, yield results which pinpoint one named medical condition or another, such as multiple sclerosis or arthritis, so that a fixed label is then attached to this condition, dictating the future treatments in terms of this label and this label only. One of the weaknesses of Western medicine, though, may be the unvarying nature of such a diagnosis, which is often belied by changes occurring over time so that this diagnosis may actually no longer hold true because other pathological changes have occurred which may alter or make invalid the original diagnosis. One of my patients, for example, had been treated for many years for a hyperactive thyroid, only to find after the onset of some cardiac condition that her thyroid function, to everybody's surprise, was now normal.

In five element acupuncture, on the other hand, we do not rely on the apparent finality of a fixed diagnosis, luckily in a way, because we have no diagnostic procedures to define the patient's element so clearly for us. We are therefore constantly aware of the uncertainties of our diagnosis, observing our patients all the time carefully for evidence that the treatment of whatever element we have chosen is having the effect we hope for, and being always prepared to amend our diagnosis if it is not. As part of this ongoing diagnosis, we have to work out for each patient our own assessment of what we hope the outcome of the treatment should be. If we are doing our work properly we are therefore constantly checking what we think our treatment should achieve with what is happening to our patient. We can certainly never sit back comfortably and rely on time-honoured treatment formulae. Each patient therefore requires an individual approach. I find the level of uncertainty and the demands this places upon me as a five element practitioner exhilarating and challenging, and have always done so. I cannot reach for a compendium of acupuncture points to help me here, as a physician can search in a drugs compendium. Others may find this too daunting, and look for branches of acupuncture which have more rigidly structured diagnostic procedures.

We must always be aware that there is the possibility of more than a slight hint of arrogance in any belief we have that we know what it is a patient needs from us. Who, indeed, are we to imagine that we understand our patient sufficiently after perhaps only a few hours with them to have what could be called the audacity to assume that we can accurately assess what their needs are? As I have stressed before, there has to be humility in all that we do, and certainly in our approach to understanding our patient. If we are to assess a patient's needs appropriately, we need time to do this, and we need constantly to test our assessment against what effect our treatment is having, each time creating a kind of reality check. Our assessment has to run parallel with what is happening in treatment. This is why I call our original diagnosis just the first step in a constantly evolving diagnostic progression. Making a diagnosis is therefore always based on putting forward a hypothesis which we must test for its validity each time the patient comes back to see us. Feedback we gain from the effect of treatment may well change our diagnosis, moving us away from one element and closer to another.

Learning how to recognise that treatment is helping our patient is a crucial area of our practice. We have to learn to train ourselves to begin to see the subtle evidence of changes to a patient's elements after treatment, which will be the start of the process by which we determine whether our treatment is proceeding as it should. This is where the sensitivity of our own senses plays such an important role, for what we are looking for is evidence of some change, however subtle. This does not necessarily involve, indeed rarely does involve, immediate changes experienced by patients themselves from the very start of treatment, but is usually a gradual overall improvement, an enhancement in general well-being, accompanied, if we are lucky, by some improvement in any physical symptoms the patient may be complaining of. These changes may not initially always be welcome to the patient, and may indeed be uncomfortable as the elements within them have to learn to adjust themselves to what is now demanded of them. We may need to warn patients of this, on the principle, which they usually understand, that things may actually have to get worse before they get better. This principle, known from homeopathy as the Law of Cure, and which five element acupuncture has incorporated into its practice, acknowledges that there may well be reactions to treatment that re-awaken some manifestation of earlier conditions, memories of which the body has retained and which the acupuncture treatment releases and then dispels.

There may be only the slightest of changes, consisting maybe of an observation that the patient looks a little different, but sometimes with no very clear sense of what exactly has changed. The patient may appear to be standing a little straighter, or looking a little less worried. Maybe we ourselves begin to feel easier in the patient's presence, as though some weight has been lifted from them, or they have started to hold our hand more easily as we take their pulses rather than gripping it tightly.

We need not strain ourselves to look for evidence of some change, but as we become more proficient we will perceive change more clearly and more quickly. I know that I now quite often notice that the shape of a patient's face has changed in some way after an Aggressive Energy (AE) drain. This may happen, surprisingly, even if there is no AE there. I attribute this to the fact that an AE drain addresses each yin official, and the contact between the needle and the acupuncture point sends a signal to each of these officials that attention is being directed at them, like a flare illuminating the sky to alert a ship in distress that help is at hand. The mother of one of my patients told her son that he looked as if he was taller after his first treatment, and measured him to prove that this was in fact so. I saw this as evidence that the relief the elements experienced after treatment was expressing itself in a relaxation of tension so that his body did indeed straighten up, and her son did walk taller.

We always have to be careful to keep our own expectations at a realistic level, since improvement as a result of acupuncture treatment will always be related to the level of imbalance in our patient. The more serious the condition, the longer treatment will take to have any effect. Our patients will be suffering from many different levels of imbalance, and over different lengths of time. Longstanding complaints of any kind will inevitably take longer to clear than something that happened only yesterday. Similarly, deeper levels of imbalance may well require longer to heal than the more superficial.

CHAPTER 20

THE OUTCOME OF TREATMENT

I think most of us assume that a successful course of treatment should result in the patient feeling better in some way. But in what way? And who decides what feeling better actually represents? In Western medical terms the successful outcome of any treatment can probably be judged as being whether the physical symptoms have improved or disappeared. But when we view things from a less physically oriented point of view, as a five element acupuncturist or a psychotherapist would do, the role physical symptoms play in assessing the success of treatment is much less clear-cut.

We take it for granted that we are offering treatment for soul as well as for body, and are therefore viewing things holistically, so how do we gauge how successful our treatment has been in helping our patient at this deeper level? This is a much more difficult question to answer than merely noting that a patient is suffering from fewer headaches or is sleeping better, and the outcome of treatment may therefore be much more difficult to assess. We then have to consider more complex questions, such as a patient's own assessment of how far treatment may have helped them in changing some more intangible aspect of their life. This could involve something like coming to terms with a past emotional trauma or having the courage to confront an unresolved issue with a partner. Improvements in these areas of life are difficult to quantify, because they are based on much more subjective criteria, and may often at first hardly be perceived by the patient and only by a practitioner trained to notice what are often very subtle changes.

I learnt a very important lesson not long ago, which has given me a different perspective on the whole issue of what can be considered a failure of treatment. A patient told me that he had been given my name 'by a friend of mine who said you had transformed her life'. I was puzzled, because I could hardly remember who this former patient was. Looking up my notes afterwards, I found that she had come for just two treatments and then disappeared. At the time I had assumed that she had not been happy with treatment, and I therefore listed her amongst those I thought I had not managed to help. Obviously, though, this was not how the patient herself had viewed things. This taught me that we can never really know how far what we have done for our patients has helped them or not, or indeed what they themselves want from treatment. It is therefore likely that patients and practitioners will have different criteria by which to judge the success or failure of treatment. It also helped me understand the importance of not becoming too self-critical, a tendency I think we all have, particularly when we start in practice, because we may not be aware that our expectations are not matching those of our patient.

We must always ask ourselves whether what we assume our patient wants from treatment is actually what they are coming to us for. Perhaps the few treatments I gave my former patient were all she felt she needed to set her life on the right path again, whilst I might have been considering a different outcome for her. The very simple but profound treatments of the Aggressive Energy drain and an element's source points which we start our treatments with can by themselves give a strong boost to the elements and help them regain balance. An AE drain, for example, is a way of asking the elements whether they have been invaded by harmful negative energy, and, if so, clearing it from the body. Addressing an element's source points is one of the deepest and safest ways of stimulating that element's energy. These first treatments therefore set the tone for all subsequent treatments, and act as their firm foundation.

Perhaps for some patients, as with my former patient, this simple treatment is all they need. Others, though, come for more than this, and may be uneasy about being left to sort out their life by themselves without ongoing support from their practitioner. If this is so, it is a clear reminder that each of us is likely to want something uniquely different from treatment, often related to the specific needs of our element, and that it is the acupuncturist's task to gauge these needs sensitively and try to satisfy them in the best way possible.

We can also waste a lot of time analysing each treatment in too much detail to see whether we could have done better. Some good advice I was given early on, which I have found increasingly easy to follow the older I get, is to stop thinking about our patients the moment they leave the practice room at the end of treatment, and not continue to clutter our minds up by taking thoughts about the first patient with us into the next patient's treatment, or home with us at the end of the day to preoccupy us later on. Originally I thought that switching off from a patient too quickly at the end of treatment might be doing them a disservice, but I now realise that the opposite is true. Before the start of each treatment, it is useful to give ourselves time to empty our minds of what has gone before so that our next patient receives the full attention from us that they need, not the half-distracted attention somebody still preoccupied with thinking about the last patient will bring them. And then when the patient comes back next time we are fully able to concentrate on them once again.

It is of course natural to continue to think through the events of our day when we have finished practising, but we should try to do this at quiet times and not during the hurly-burly of the day's activities. Only then can we clear our minds sufficiently to help us sort out any problems we need to deal with. All this is easier said than done, but if we are aware of some of the issues which make practising problematic for us, we are halfway to solving them.

CHAPTER 21

WE CAN FALL INTO BAD HABITS

We can fall into bad habits over the years, becoming careless in what we do. One such pitfall is that we may become a little bit too comfortable in our work, and do not challenge ourselves as much as we should. We may start to forget that each time we see our patient we see a slightly different person who is altered by the passage of time, and therefore that the patient before us is never the same as the person we saw at the last treatment. We have to understand the need to look at them with fresh eyes, requiring possibly a different approach from us.

It is indeed very difficult to retain a freshness of approach to our patients if they have been coming to us for a long time. Often we are only too pleased to welcome patients we think are doing well, because we feel they are unlikely to challenge us by presenting us with new problems. These are patients whose treatment we assume to know in advance. Here we can be at risk of falling into rather too well-worn a rut if we are not careful, thinking that our patients will be as they were before. Perhaps unconsciously we ignore the possibility that they may have changed in some way, since changes require us to make more effort. It is much easier, we may think, to continue doing what we have done so apparently satisfactorily before.

And then we may not see, or choose not to see, something in our patient which should be pointing us in a new direction. A long-term patient of mine, whose treatment I regarded as being simple to plan ahead for, turned up for one appointment not as I expected her to be. If I had not been alert I could easily have overlooked the slight change I perceived in her. She herself volunteered nothing until I probed a little more and discovered that quite a disturbing event had happened to her, which totally changed the direction of the treatment I was intending to give. Looking back on this afterwards I realised that I had been in danger of assuming in advance that I would find her as I had done before, and might perhaps have ignored the pointer alerting me to a need to re-evaluate the treatment I was intending to give her, which was now no longer appropriate.

We must never assume that we know our patient's needs of today, since yesterday may have changed them.

CHAPTER 22

NOT DEMANDING TOO MUCH OF OURSELVES

It is also very important that all five element acupuncturists, particularly those in the early stages of their practice, do not burden themselves unduly with unnecessarily high expectations of their own sensory skills. It takes many years to develop them, and for different people one or other of the four classical diagnostic skills of hearing, seeing, smelling and feeling will always be easier to acquire than the others. Some of these sensory skills may, indeed, remain stubbornly inaccessible to us even after many years trying to hone them. It is good to work out early in our practice which of these we may have a particular affinity for, and base our diagnosis predominantly on this whilst waiting for our other senses to catch up over time.

At the heart of good practice lies one of many simple lessons. We must never assume that our skills, whether diagnostic, such as in our ability to pinpoint sensory information correctly, or interpersonal, such as in our ability to relate appropriately to our patients, are as acute as we may like to think they are. There must always be an element of self-questioning in all aspects of our practice, a refusal to accept things as self-evident so that we are forced constantly to be on the alert in case what we may have assumed is so ('this voice is weeping', 'this smell is fragrant', 'this emotion is joy') may not in fact be so at all. Instead, as we will often find, it may simply be the most strident expression of one of the elements which is actually disguising the true element in distress. A very obvious mistake, for example, is the failure to see fear (coming from the Water element) hiding behind a slightly hysterical expression of joy (which is thought to come from the Fire element). And there have been many times when I have been pulled up short by discovering that what had to me 'obviously' been a sign of a particular element was, just as obviously once I had recognised it, that of quite a different element.

How then do we track these elusive things, the elements, down so that eventually we make the right choice? Always it is a matter of giving ourselves the necessary time and patience not to become either disheartened or too over-eager so that we snatch at the first sign an element may be giving us without waiting for further, deeper confirmation that what we think is so is truly so. We are often so relieved to have discovered what we believe to be a clear sign of an element's presence in our patient that we may allow it to dazzle us too soon into thinking that we have found the true element, and draw back our horns as it were, by stopping just there and not really looking any further.

CHAPTER 23

NOBODY LIKES GETTING THINGS WRONG

One of the most difficult lessons for a five element acupuncturist is learning to train ourselves not to mind if our choice of element eventually turns out not to be the 'right' one. I can still remember my feeling of embarrassment when the whole of my Leamington class except for me thought a patient was quite clearly Earth, when I was sure she was Metal. I remember cringing inside when I realised that there was something in the patient which I had not before then associated with Earth, but everybody else had, and my shame at having to admit this in front of the 20 or so of my fellow students.

I have often baulked at using the words 'right' and 'wrong' when talking about the elements, because these terms hide within them just this feeling I had in the class of not being good enough, or at least of not being as good as other people. But there is definitely a 'right' element, which is the patient's element, and eventually 'wrong' elements, which are the four other elements that are not this patient's element. We have to learn to accept, though, that discovering the right element always takes a lot of time and a lot of experience, but does not come as a result of a flash of insight in a few moments. It helps to know that the cumulative experience of years of practice undoubtedly speeds this process up.

I have tried to think of better ways of describing an element as being either the 'right' or the 'wrong' one, but have not yet come up with any satisfactory alternative. So these descriptions may have to stay, despite making us feel just as inadequate as we felt at school when we got an answer in class wrong. 'Not yet the right element' is the nearest I have come to a possible solution, but although it is an accurate description of the step-by-step process of diagnosis it does not slip easily from the tongue. Perhaps with more frequent use, though, it will gradually start to supersede the phrase 'the wrong element' with all its unhappy associations.

I have often thought that this is one of the reasons why people hesitate to venture into five element acupuncture. Other branches of acupuncture seem to display their diagnostic choices in less black and white terms, and can therefore seem to expose their practitioners less to public displays of what they may wrongly feel as their ignorance.

Significantly though, this, to me, embarrassing lesson in not recognising the Earth element taught me the most I have ever learnt about Earth in the shortest time. As JR Worsley would tell us: 'You don't learn anything if you get the element right. It's when you get it wrong that you learn the most.'

CHAPTER 24

More on the Patient– Practitioner Relationship

What I did not realise to start with in relation to my teaching in China was something which I take very much for granted in my teaching in Europe. And I learnt a lot from a very illuminating incident at one of my earliest seminars which surprised me. I happened to be staying in the same hotel as some of the course participants, and greeted a few of them in the hotel lobby. At the end of the seminar when I asked them to tell me what they had learnt, one of them burst into tears and said that she had been overwhelmed by meeting me in the hotel on her first day. I asked her why this was, and she said, 'You looked at me.' Afterwards I tried to think whether there had been anything special about my greeting of her, but could only recall smiling at her as we said hello to each other. But I made eye contact with her as I do with everybody I greet, and, I suppose, warm eye contact, because I was really pleased to meet some of the people coming to the seminar. Eye contact of this kind, I then realised, must have been something new to her.

That made me ask myself what I do as I greet somebody, so I observed myself a little more to see if I could gauge why the kind of eye contact I made with her had surprised and moved her. I went on to compare what I observed about myself in my interaction with others with how I saw people greeting each other in China. When the students greeted each other, they did so just as warmly as similar groups would do in this country, but I noticed that the interactions of the course participants with senior tutors were very different. The students would scuttle past with their heads lowered as if they were trying to get out of the way as soon as possible.

I then thought about how I myself was treated in China when in the company of other professional people. The most obvious example of this came from an occasion when I formed part of a group of senior professionals who were invited to sit on the platform at a conference. The group waited together in a side-room before being led out. To my surprise none of the other people in the room looked at me or made any attempt to engage with me in any way at all, although they talked a little amongst themselves. At one point, just before being led out into the auditorium, I was standing within a few feet of somebody to whom I had been introduced on another occasion, and turned to smile at him, as I would naturally do. I felt rebuffed as he refused to make eye contact with me, looking fixedly at a point to my side. A similar thing happened on several other occasions, until it dawned on me that personal contact of this kind was not acceptable between people of some seniority, and therefore also presumably between tutors and students. Hence the young woman's surprise at my warm greeting in the hotel.

This observation fed into my thoughts on how Chinese acupuncturists greet their own patients, and how far removed this is from the very warm personal relationship I have with my own patients and have taught all my students to develop with theirs. This made me more aware of the fact that a common concern for Chinese participants was that they felt that their training had not equipped them to enter into any relationship with their patients, apart from asking them to list their physical complaints. As an elderly practitioner told me sadly, 'I watch you talking to the patients. I don't know how to start talking to them like that.'

This made me gradually realise that underlying the very different approach to patients we offer and the Chinese acupuncturists were trained to offer lay a vast cultural divide which I would somehow have to address if my teaching was to be productive. So how did I do this? Mostly by using myself as an example of how to approach patients. One patient after another would sit with me in front of the class, and I would then engage with them in the way I would if I was alone with them in my practice room in London. Of course the situation was very far from the same. I had to train myself to try to ignore the row upon row of those watching. Nothing can, of course, replicate the calm atmosphere we try to create for our patients in our own practice, but I had to do the best that I could. I honestly don't now know how successful I am in doing this. I know, though, that with experience I have learnt increasingly to blank out the presence of all those watching me, and concentrate only on the patient.

There is always the added difficulty that each word spoken by the patient has to be translated for me, and each word I speak to the patient has to be translated back to them, and even if the patient can speak English, the questions and replies have to be translated for all the class to understand. Inevitably this holds up the flow of my interaction with a patient. What has offset this difficulty a little, though, is the fact that the practitioners presenting their patients to the class before the patients arrive have learnt to give their presentations so well in imitation of what they have watched me do that what they say about their patients now also covers in great detail their patients' emotional lives and the stresses they are experiencing. This is testament to how much these practitioners have learnt from each of the seminars they have attended.

Initially they would simply recite a long list of the patient's physical complaints, with no attempt to place the patient in any context, such as their family or work situation, or any problems they might be experiencing. Physical symptoms were paramount, and what was going on emotionally was not touched upon. To start with they found it difficult to change their mind-set. Watching me questioning patients about all aspects of their lives was therefore rather startling for them, and it took some time for them to dare approach this area. But they learnt surprisingly quickly, and were eager to venture on to unfamiliar emotional terrain. Now, I am delighted to see how well they have taken on board what they have observed from my interactions with patients.

This soon made me aware of another aspect of my work. Patients in this country are so familiar with psychological therapies of all kinds that most patients are not at all taken aback to find their acupuncturist asking them about the stresses in their life, taking it almost for granted that these have an effect upon their bodies. The same does not hold true in China, where there has so far been much less emphasis, not to say no emphasis at all, on the effects of psychological stress and its relationship to ill health.

With therapies like acupuncture, and in particular in this respect five element acupuncture with its emphasis on the emotional aspects of the elements, the wholeness of the human being and thus the importance of continuing to link body and soul together in whatever area of health we are working is paramount and self-evident. In modern Chinese medicine, on the other hand, this is not the case, perhaps surprisingly, since the importance of the human being forming an indivisible whole of body and soul is clearly stated in the classical texts which all acupuncturists learn by heart during their training and on which they still base their practice. As modern China started to re-evaluate its approach to health and its own traditional medicine, and with it succumbed to the dominating influence of what was regarded as an utterly modern and therefore much to be emulated branch of medicine, that of Western medicine, it began to take on Western medicine's emphasis on the purely physical basis of all disease. Traditional medicine, based on apparently archaic, scientifically unproven principles, was made to give way to this new approach.

The more elusive qualities of Chinese traditional medicine then came increasingly to be regarded as outdated and old-fashioned. It is ironic then that it has been the appreciation of just those qualities which the modern Chinese world felt slightly ashamed of, a spiritual approach to the human being in health and ill health, which have proved attractive to the Western world, and encouraged it to explore China's traditional medicine, and then slowly to take it to its heart. This, in turn, has influenced how the Chinese view their own indigenous medicine. The two strands of Chinese medicine, the physical and the psychological which were originally fused together in former times, having become disconnected through contact with Western medicine, have now started to draw together again, as Western medicine discovers that it, too, cannot just shrug of the psychological aspects of ill health by trying to belittle it with such words as the placebo effect. Nor can the undoubted effectiveness of acupuncture as a healing discipline over several millennia be waved away as somehow scientifically unverifiable and therefore insignificant. After all nobody knows how aspirin works, and yet we know it relieves pain. All the more so we can see that, though the mechanisms by which acupuncture needles stimulate points on the body and thereby effect a return to health at all levels are not scientifically understood, their effectiveness cannot be denied.

PART 4

Teaching Other Practitioners

CHAPTER 25

THE COURAGE TO BECOME A FIVE ELEMENT ACUPUNCTURIST

A practitioner told me that she knew that many of her fellow practitioners, trained as she had originally been in TCM, were trying to study five element acupuncture with the idea of practising it, but were too timid to start incorporating it into their practice without more help because they felt too uncertain about diagnosing the elements. Unlike them, this practitioner had had the courage to take the difficult step of changing over to a pure five element approach to practice, because she knew that this was where her heart really lay.

This set me thinking about whether there was something here which I need to incorporate more into my teaching plans. It seems to me that there is a great need to work out ways of demystifying five element acupuncture, so that we can help people to be less afraid of venturing on to a five element landscape in their practice, as this practitioner's friends are. I often feel that a kind of aura seems to hang over five element practice for those unfamiliar with it, and this is a preconception I have tried to dispel. Five element practitioners accept as a given that their discipline approaches the deeper aspects of the psyche, as well as its physical envelope, the body. With appropriate training this is not something which needs to be thought of as disturbing, but should rather be seen as making our practice so rewarding. It may, however, be one of the reasons why those from other acupuncture disciplines which lay less emphasis, or sometimes none at all, upon these deeper aspects of human experience may find it too daunting because they are asked to explore areas which are unfamiliar to them. Hence their quite natural reluctance to challenge themselves by doing so.

I ask myself how I can best help those people who are so keen to learn and ask for support, particularly now when, for many reasons, there are few experienced five element acupuncturists prepared to teach. To understand this better I have been examining in detail what I would regard as the components of an ideal approach to learning five element acupuncture.

Perhaps the most important aspect is an intense curiosity about human nature as expressing itself in the practitioner themselves and in all those they encounter, patients and people in everyday life alike. You have to want to explore what makes the human being tick if you are going to set yourself on the path to help others in this discipline. Direct experience of life in all its ups and down (and the downs teach us more than the ups) is therefore a necessary pre-condition for setting out on a five element path.

Obviously, from its name alone, we know that the elements form the bedrock of what we do, and the only way to start learning about how the elements reveal themselves in each one of us is to use our different senses as we encounter one person after another. We also need to have the necessary humility to study ourselves with honesty. The five element mantra teaches us that we need to look for the signs which the different senses imprint upon us. We need to learn to use our eyes to perceive things more accurately, our noses to smell things more acutely, our ears to hear things more clearly and our emotional antennae to detect the emotional presence of the elements more sensitively in all we meet. There is unfortunately no short-cut available to us here. It always takes time to develop the increasingly sophisticated sensory apparatus within ourselves which will eventually guide us to a correct diagnosis of the different elements, and help us pinpoint the one in particular, the one I call the guardian element and JR Worsley called the element of the causative factor of disease (the CF), on which our treatment will be focused. We cannot rely upon others to tell us what they are seeing, hearing, smelling and feeling, because we have to develop our own senses. And we also have to learn that this takes time, a lot of time. We often start by thinking that it is not as difficult as people tell us, and make rather rash judgements which can often prove wrong. I can well remember that I did this, and had to learn to cultivate greater humility and patience. Now, much wiser and older, I never say that I 'know' what a patient's element is, but only that 'I think the element is...', until treatment confirms my diagnosis.

With experience we accumulate our own sensory templates for the individual elements, which we add to with each patient treated successfully. Of course we are helped to do this by learning from other more experienced practitioners, but at some point we have to dare venture on our own, remembering that the first encounter with a new patient is always taking us to an unknown place. We may be lucky enough to have one or more senses which are more highly developed than others. I remember that one of my fellow students at acupuncture college was very sensitive to smell, and could diagnose this very accurately. In my case, even now I seem to concentrate more on how a patient makes me feel, in other words on the emotional aspect of my relationship with them, than on my other senses, although these will also at different times help direct my treatments towards one or other element, sometimes unexpectedly. A sound suddenly heard in a patient's voice may startle me and guide me towards a different element than the one I am concentrating upon. The colour on a patient's body, perhaps contrasting itself with that of my own skin as I place my hand on the patient's arm, may set my thoughts moving in another direction. I can feel myself surprised into thinking, 'Goodness, I think this may be Wood after all' rather than another element I initially thought it might be.

Humility, the need never to be too proud to change one's mind or to admit that one really doesn't know, is an absolutely essential quality we all have to develop. For some people, this sense of the ultimate unknowability of another person leads them into dangerous areas they would prefer to avoid. For those who want certainty as they work, five element acupuncture is not for them, since deep within each human being is something ultimately mysterious, often unknowable even to themselves. Of course it can seem easier and less challenging to look up in a book what points to use today when the tongue is a certain colour, than to venture into the unknown, as we have to do. In my view, we cannot really help another person, at whatever level, whether of body or soul, unless we are aware of this.

I have been watching some lovely BBC programmes on Japan at the moment, to coincide with a major exhibition on the artist, Hokusai, he of the great wave. Amongst many other interesting insights I was delighted to hear the following: 'The Japanese worship the unknowable. The answer is not the point. It is a search that will never end. That's why we value the unknowable': this from a Zen Buddhist priest. The Japanese, I was told, 'embrace the beauty of mystery'. Five element acupuncturists, too, have to be prepared to do just that.

And then Hokusai apparently said the following, as though with me in mind, I felt:

> From the age of six I had the desire to copy the form of things.
>
> ...
>
> But until the age of 70, nothing I drew was worthy of notice.
> At the age of 73 I was somewhat able to fathom the growth of plants and trees, and the structure of birds and animals, insects and fish.
> Then when I reach 80 years I hope to have made increasing progress
> And at 90 to see further into the underlying principle of things,
> So that at 100 years I will have achieved the divine state in my art
> And then at 110 every dot and every stroke will be as though alive.[1]

I like to think that at 80 years I am making 'increasing progress' in my acupuncture practice and in my thoughts on acupuncture, so that at 90 I will be able to 'see further into the underlying principle of things'. If I have the good luck to reach 100 how nice it would be to think that, like Hokusai, 'I will have achieved the divine state in my art' as acupuncturist. One hundred and ten seems unfortunately too far off, but perhaps in whatever sphere of existence I am then, maybe 'every dot and every stroke' of my writings will still 'be as though alive'.

And finally, the programme on Hokusai ended with a lovely clip of David Hockney saying:

> The Chinese say you need three things for painting: the hand, the eye and the heart. Two won't do.

---

1   Katsushika Hokusai in Wheatley, P. (dir.) (2017) *Hokusai. Old Man Crazy to Paint.* BBC 4.

I think you can say exactly the same about acupuncture.
We definitely need the hand and the eye, but it is the heart
which completes us. Two only definitely won't do.

CHAPTER 26

THE LACK OF TEACHERS

I am a little puzzled when I look at the present position which five element acupuncture occupies in this country's acupuncture scene. I have written before about the rather surprisingly antagonistic approach to five element acupuncture which developed just as I completed my advanced studies under JR Worsley. I am glad to see that this shadow is gradually starting to dissipate, not least, I like to think, because of the growing interest in five element acupuncture now being shown in China itself which has taken it to its heart in a way and with such speed that perhaps none of us could have foreseen. Certainly I could not, as I began the series of five element seminars there some six years ago.

The problem, though, is that the growing Chinese enthusiasm for learning five element acupuncture is increasingly coming up against the lack of experienced five element practitioners prepared to teach. One of the hurdles here is that there are now so few practitioners who practise only five element acupuncture, and only these can be considered to have sufficient experience to teach.

If a practitioner's training has not given them the opportunity to explore the nature of the different elements in sufficient depth and over a sufficiently long period of time, they will have difficulty gaining enough confidence in their diagnostic skills to practise five element acupuncture when they graduate. This is what many students emerging from these combined courses have told me; they often do not know where to turn to find five element practitioners with sufficient experience to help them gain the confidence they need.

To encourage people who may consider teaching at some point I have many times told them what JR Worsley said to me when I expressed my doubts about my right to teach others, and I repeat here: 'Remember, Nora, you know more than they do.' The only quality a proficient teacher must have is to accept that they know a little more than those they are teaching, and not to be frightened of saying that they do not know more than they do. It certainly does not mean that they have to know a lot more than their students, and certainly not that they need to claim to know everything. Indeed good teachers never claim that. I have always recognised that I can learn only from those who are prepared to say when they do not know something. JR Worsley would acknowledge if a student had a new thought which had not occurred to him, as he did once with me, to my surprise and delight.

We have to be humble as practitioners, and even more humble, I feel, as teachers. The kind of humility which is prepared to acknowledge in front of a class of students that it doesn't know the answer to a student's question demands a lot of courage from a teacher. At heart we would all like our students to admire us as people who have an answer to everything. The reality, though, is quite different. Life always contains an element of the unknowable, and our students are often there to teach us this.

CHAPTER 27

ADAPTING TO A CHINESE CONTEXT

Initially I was very unclear what was demanded of me in China. Those who invited me, principally Liu Lihong, were also not sure what the exact purpose of my visit was. Was I there to show Chinese acupuncturists the broad outlines of what five element acupuncture was about and the kind of treatment I gave as a five element acupuncturist, a kind of theoretical introduction to its principles? Or was I there to teach practitioners how to incorporate five element acupuncture into their practice? It dawned on me very soon that it was going to be entirely up to me how I was going to define the purpose and scope of my visits, and I have continued to learn on the job, as it were, each visit modifying slightly what we have done before. Each seminar therefore develops a new approach which is demanded by the increasing sophistication of the five element practice which our very keen and very professional Chinese acupuncturists are engaged in.

It was clear from the start that there was great curiosity about the unfamiliar approach to acupuncture which five element acupuncture represented. The ground had been well prepared in advance by Liu Lihong, first by a visit to him from Mei Long, now a fellow tutor of mine at my Chinese seminars. She lives in the Netherlands, and in 2010 she attended a seminar I gave there. She told me about somebody called Professor Liu Lihong who had written an immensely popular book, *Classical Chinese*

Medicine,[1] which has for years been on the bestseller lists in China. Having read this book and knowing about Liu Lihong's strong feeling that there needs to be a different approach to traditional medicine in China, Mei wrote an impassioned letter to him making him aware of the existence of a branch of traditional medicine which echoed deeply Liu Lihong's own beliefs. She felt that five element acupuncture represented an important re-connection to the principles of traditional medicine which Liu Lihong felt so strongly about.

As a result of this letter she was invited to his research institute, the Tongyou Sanhe centre in Nanning, to give a series of introductory talks on five element acupuncture. These talks stimulated very great interest, and led to my meeting Liu Lihong at a conference in Rothenburg, and to his inviting me to give another seminar in Nanning. At the same time, Mei set about translating my book, *The Handbook of Five Element Practice*[2] into Mandarin as a first step to introducing five element acupuncture back to China.

She and I held our first seminar in Nanning in October 2011, which was the start of the twice-yearly visits we have made since then. Each seminar we have given has led to our teaching an ever increasing body of very dedicated five element acupuncturists, many of whom are themselves now teaching others.

The small team from Europe, consisting initially only of Mei and me, was joined a few seminars later by Guy Caplan, a former graduate of SOFEA. The three of us form the core teaching team in China, with an increasing amount of work now happily delegated to a group of the

---

1   Lihong, L. (2003) *Sikao Zhongyi: Classical Chinese Medicine*. Hong Kong: The Chinese University Press.
2   Franglen, N. (2014) *The Handbook of Five Element Practice*. London: Singing Dragon.

most experienced Chinese five element acupuncturists themselves. This group has now taken over the running of introductory courses which are held in various towns in China as preparation for our seminars. Those we teach have therefore passed beyond the elementary stage, making it possible for our work to move on to the more advanced level. This means that at each visit we are teaching increasingly experienced five element practitioners. What simplifies our task is that all those attending are already qualified acupuncturists with a thorough training in the rudiments of acupuncture, such as needling and point location.

Of course, Guy and I are handicapped by not speaking Mandarin, which is where Mei as a native speaker provides some light relief when she teaches in her mother tongue. Our hosts get round the problem of our teaching in English beautifully by allocating to each of us a dedicated translator who sticks closely to our sides wherever we go, as we pass from lecture room to practice room. Many more of the participants understand English than they confess to, but are inhibited from speaking it. I know this because when I make a joke or laugh, as I often like to do to lighten the atmosphere in the classroom and relax the students, more people laugh before hearing the translation than I expect them to. And more people want to buy copies of my books in their English editions than, again, I would expect them to if their knowledge of English was inadequate.

CHAPTER 28

WHY I ENJOY TEACHING IN CHINA SO MUCH

I often ask myself why I enjoy teaching so much in China and why this is so different from the teaching I do in this country or in Europe. The answer I always give people who also ask me this is that I find it easier, and, to that extent, more satisfying for many reasons. The most obvious, superficial reason may well be the way I am welcomed over there, which is as a revered visitor. This is so unlike how students in this country treat their teachers, where the approach is much more irreverent than reverent. In China the reverse is true; there the culture is built on a deep respect for tradition, and for their teachers who embody this.

Through one of the serendipities of life (oh how I love that word!), I happen now to be reading a book called *The Souls of China: The Return of Religion after Mao*[1] (yes, souls, not soul!) by Ian Johnson. Here are some brief extracts:

> Faith and values are returning to the centre of a national discussion over how to organise Chinese life... As one person I interviewed for this book told me, 'We thought we were unhappy because we were poor. But now a lot of us aren't poor anymore, and yet we're still unhappy. We realise there's something missing and that's a spiritual life.' (pp.16–17)

---

1 Johnson, I. (2017) *The Souls of China: The Return of Religion after Mao.* London: Allen Lane.

All told, it is hardly an exaggeration to say China is undergoing a spiritual revival similar to the Great Awakening in the United States in the nineteenth century. Now, just like a century and a half ago, a country on the move is unsettled by great social and economic change. People have been thrust into new, alienating cities where they have no friends and no circle of support. Religion and faith offer ways of looking at age-old questions that all people, everywhere, struggle to answer: Why are we here? What really makes us happy? How do we achievement contentment as individuals, as a community, as a nation? What is our soul? (pp.17–18)

This reminds me of something the administrator of a large Chinese province told me as I was treating him. To my surprise, he said, 'We need you in China, Nora laoshi (Teacher Nora). We have lost our soul.' My surprise was that the person saying this was a provincial administrator, not, as one might expect, a practitioner of some spiritual discipline. I smiled when I thought to myself how incongruous such a statement would sound coming from his British equivalent, a politician or a banker. What it confirmed for me was the essential spiritual nature which lies deep within the Chinese character, and it is partly this which explains much of the satisfaction I experience in my teaching over there.

For I regard five element acupuncture as a form of spiritual practice, not merely as a purely physical medical discipline. It is that, too, of course, but it is much more than this, and it is this 'more' which first attracted me to it, and keeps me so firmly enthralled by it that I cannot see myself abandoning my practice until my knees will no longer keep me upright and my hands shake too much to hold a needle. Today, for example, I was faced with the need to help a longstanding patient of mine whose partner of many years had suddenly left without forewarning, leaving her devastated. I cast around a little in my mind trying to think of what treatment I could choose to help her, but hardly had I taken her pulses when I was suddenly struck by the thought that, of course, these were the circumstances which were most likely to create what is known as a Husband/Wife imbalance. The pulses themselves had not at first suggested this, so subtle can be the signs of this imbalance, and, as I often say, how crude and clumsy will always be our pulse-taking in the face of the very delicate nature of the pulses.

But the situation obviously pointed to a classic Husband/Wife situation (relationship problems being typical evidence for this imbalance), and though I wasn't initially convinced that I was interpreting the pulse picture accurately, I decided to carry out the procedure. The result confirmed what I had guessed might be there. The patient's pulses steadied themselves beautifully after treatment, and as she left she said, 'I feel quite different. When I came I felt I couldn't cope, now I feel more hopeful that I will be able to deal with this.' I am making sure that she comes for a further treatment within a week, as one should always do in such cases. After all, this indicates an attack upon the Heart, which will remain vulnerable for some time and needs regular strengthening to prevent the block returning.

For me, the experience of treating my patient was akin to a spiritual experience. The atmosphere in the practice room, from start to finish, reflected something deeply emotional. Long after the patient left, this feeling persisted in me. We were, after all, both in our different ways facing a situation of profound crisis, and I was being asked to help my patient at the deepest level. Sometimes one hears the most beautiful sayings which illuminate one's day quite by chance. On the radio yesterday I heard Archbishop Sentamu, the Archbishop of York, a really gentle, caring man, say, 'We do not have a window into people's souls.' But even though I agree that I did not have a window into my patient of today's soul, I felt that my treatment had allowed a little more healing light to stream into that window hidden deep within her.

This spiritual dimension of my work, and the fact that this is immediately understood by Chinese practitioners, is one of the main reasons why teaching in China is such a satisfactory experience for me. Since the basic components of my work, such as the Dao, yin yang and the five elements, are familiar to every Chinese person, this makes it very easy for them to start to incorporate the principles of five element acupuncture into their practice. No longer do I need to answer the kind of questions my students in England would ask me with a puzzled air, such as, 'How do we know that there are things called elements?', or 'What evidence is there for the existence of acupuncture points?' These are both perfectly reasonable questions for those not brought up in an environment where the elements perfuse every strand of everyday life, and where to cast doubt on the existence of acupuncture points and the efficacy of acupuncture itself could be considered futile and almost sacrilegious in the strict meaning of the word (an affront to a basically religious belief). To embark on the task of introducing an understanding of the practice of five element acupuncture to the Chinese is akin to sowing seeds in already well-fertilised ground.

My conviction that what I practise represents a profound truth therefore receives welcome confirmation each time I set foot on Chinese soil. There I am amongst people all of whom at some deep level speak the same spiritual language I do, even if we differ in the superficial everyday languages we speak.

And how I continue to wish I could learn to understand and speak this lovely language to a level which would make proper communication possible.

CHAPTER 29

THE SIGNIFICANCE OF MY TEACHING IN CHINA

It is only in the past year that I have become aware of the significance of my work in China. When I first went there five years ago I had no inkling of the acupuncture environment I would find myself transported to. I am amazed now to think how little prepared I must have been, although, looking back from my present standpoint, perhaps this was all to the good. My mind was a completely empty slate on which the cumulative experiences gained from each visit there (now having completed my 12th) gradually wrote their own story, and one that was very different from those of my previous experiences. I now accept that it was an unexpected bonus to be as naïve as I was about what was expected of me in China, and the significance of my finding myself there at this particular stage of my life. I did not know what to expect and, to start with, I responded to what was asked of me with the sole aim of repaying my hosts for their generous welcome. It was only gradually, as I learnt to understand more about the current position of acupuncture in the Chinese medical world, that I began to adapt my teaching to take account of what I felt this position demanded of me.

That a by-product of this should have changed something very fundamental in my view of myself, particularly of myself as teacher of five element acupuncture, was not something I could possibly have foreseen. Nor could I have foreseen that the steady pressure upon me of my Chinese experiences should gradually have given me a more realistic appreciation of my own value as acupuncturist, and, by extension, also of my value as a human being, which before I might have shrugged off if it had not been reinforced so strongly at each visit to China. Perhaps until now I have never given myself an appropriate level of credit for what I have achieved in acupuncture terms both in this country and more recently in China, being the kind of person who has always been unsure of her own achievements and her position in the pecking order of life. It has therefore taken all these visits to China for me only very recently to have begun to have a deeper understanding of quite how important these visits have been, and increasingly continue to be, as part of the role I am playing in re-kindling interest in the approach to classical acupuncture which five element acupuncture represents.

Thinking about this deeply for some time now, I found myself drawn to read again the very illuminating introduction which Heiner Fruehauf has written to his forthcoming translation[1] of Professor Liu Lihong's seminal book, *Classical Chinese Medicine*. As Heiner puts it, Liu Lihong's work:

> has made this book a bestseller that is read not only by medical students and doctors in China, but by multiple strata of the general population who long for a state of health and well-being founded in a deeper sense of cultural identity. Most importantly, Prof. Liu's ardent appeal to regard Chinese medicine as a science in its own right has inspired a mainland grassroots movement that is beginning to draw talented students to a field that was long regarded as a bleak 2nd rate destination for professional development. (p.1)

---

1   Fruehauf, H. *Draft Introduction to Classical Chinese Medicine.* Portland, OR: National University of Natural Medicine.

No longer could we say that following a calling as an acupuncturist could be regarded in China as a 'bleak 2nd-rate destination'. Quite the contrary, traditional Chinese medicine is now beginning to be seen, even by the mainstream Chinese acupuncture world, as offering something particularly appropriate for a modern China increasingly aware of how the upheavals of the past 50 years have affected its approach to traditional medicine. Appropriately for their growing interest in five element acupuncture, the Chinese regard traditional acupuncture as being one of the few disciplines in China with an unbroken history, and in that lies its significance for the China of today. This, too, is the significance of my own work in China through my seminars on five element acupuncture. Against a background in which there is growing appreciation of the heritage of the past, where so much of that past has been physically and emotionally destroyed, its traditional medicine, though initially somewhat atrophied, is now sending out increasingly vigorous shoots, as the appreciation of the value of this unbroken medical lineage grows with each year that passes.

My appearance in China, with its emphasis on a practice basing itself very firmly on its classical roots with hardly a nod to Western medicine, is a re-affirmation of the validity of the fundamental principles which the modern practice of traditional acupuncture can draw from its deep past. This traditional discipline was originally weakened in China by the growing influx and often stifling influence of Western medicine, from the time of the earliest Christian missionaries onwards to the present day, accompanied as this was, and still remains for many, by the belief that this more modern medical discipline deserves greater respect than China's age-old indigenous tradition. What five element acupuncture brings to this mix is proof that the principles of this more than two-thousand-year-old system of medicine are just as valid today as they have always been throughout the ages, and are, indeed, particularly relevant when faced with the problems, both physical and emotional, of the modern world.

For five element acupuncture is admirably suited to address the needs of the individual, so often now overwhelmed by the complexities of modern life. It acknowledges the fundamental need for each of us to learn to express our individuality, whilst living socially amongst countless numbers of others equally intent on satisfying their own legitimate needs. This is foreshadowed in the earliest days of traditional acupuncture in the great compendium of Chinese medical thought, the Neijing Suwen, which clearly acknowledges the primacy and importance of the development of the individual, and expresses this in terms of the balance of the five elements within each one of us.

One of the problems in incorporating these ancient, time-proven tenets into the world of modern medicine has been the importance which the modern Chinese medical world has so far attached to seeing how far its acupuncture practice can be seen to adhere to as many of the tenets of Western medicine as possible. In effect, the tendency has been to measure traditional medicine against the precepts of Western medicine, the latter being regarded as the touchstone of how any modern medical discipline should be judged. For many years now much of modern acupuncture has therefore turned its attention westwards looking for as many areas as possible which bring it closer to orthodox Western medicine, thereby, it is often felt, lending it greater credibility in a modern world in which the scientific likes to think that is has ruled supreme until now. The idea that what cannot be scientifically proven is either valueless, or definitely has less value than what can submit itself to scientific proof means that science has spread its tentacles over many other different branches of medicine, and where these diverge from orthodox Western medical principles it attempts to bury them beneath a great blanket of scepticism. Luckily, advances in scientific knowledge have spread doubt over exactly how objective any knowledge we gain is, and this uncertainty has reached over into traditional healing arts, such as acupuncture, allowing them to emerge, not quite intact, but more intact than before, from behind the previously obscure smokescreens the Western medical world thought fit to erect to shield itself from the often uncomfortable facts which such practices made them confront.

When I say 'not quite intact', this is because unfortunately Western scepticism about acupuncture's efficacy has put its stamp on much current acupuncture training, both in the West and in China, often imbuing its practitioners with a kind of fear, so that they are reluctant to accept that traditional Chinese medicine should be regarded as a discipline complete in itself, as I believe it should, preferring instead to leave loopholes through which Western medical concepts are allowed, indeed often even encouraged, to creep into the practice of traditional acupuncture. It is as though people are hedging their bets so that they can always retreat, when challenged, into what they regard as the safety of Western medicine. It astonishes me, though, that many years after acupuncture has made its way into mainstream medical practice in the West, the need to maintain greater links to Western medicine than the practice of traditional acupuncture requires is still so strong.

And this, I think, has much to do with the difficulties experienced in trying to integrate traditional Chinese medicine into modern China's mainstream medical structure. The history of traditional medicine's emergence as a major component of modern Chinese medicine over the past 50 years is testament to some confusion as to where exactly to place its indigenous medicine. Is it a coherent system with its own inherent value, proved over thousands of years, or is it merely a blow-back to some primitive form of medical practice not appropriate for the 21st century? This confusion has become more acute as the Western world has taken China's traditional medicine increasingly to heart, openly extolling its efficacy over many years, even to the extent that acupuncture is now often recommended by orthodox medical practitioners as an effective form of treatment for various conditions. If the West, imbued for the past century or two with absolute trust in the developments of Western medicine, is now able to accept that there may be other branches of medicine that have some validity, such as traditional Chinese medicine with its thousand-year-old practices, how then should the Chinese medical world view its own traditional practices? Striving always to match its achievements with the best that the West can offer, it is beginning to realise that here is one area in which the West can look to it as having equal knowledge, indeed in some instances superior.

What makes me lay claim to the superiority of traditional Chinese acupuncture over some areas of Western medical practice is one fundamental principle underlying all that I do as a five element acupuncturist, and that is my absolute conviction that every needle I insert into an acupuncture point, an apparently physical instrument into an apparently physical object, a person's body, is not merely attempting to stimulate a person's energy at what appears obviously to be the physical level, but is also, and in my view more importantly, stimulating energy at those deeper levels of a human being, our inner world, the two, the body and the soul within that body, being always understood by traditional Chinese medicine to be one and indivisible.

This is where Western medicine lags behind its ancient Chinese counterpart, for along the path leading to its many discoveries it discarded some of its earlier understanding, deeming some ideas to be antiquated and irrelevant when viewed from a modern scientific standpoint. Thus the former understanding of illnesses as having a strong relationship to a patient's emotional constitution, which underpinned the concepts of the humours (choleric, sanguine, etc.), was soon rejected as formulating a primitive approach to health in the light of scientific advances which placed the physical at the forefront of all its attention. What existed deep inside a person, which previously had had equal, if not sometimes greater, diagnostic importance, disappeared from view, only re-appearing, but in attenuated form, in recent years under the concept of psychosomatic conditions, often spoken of in somewhat disparaging terms as somehow being less worthy of attention than purely physical symptoms. The world of the body has taken centre stage in all Western medical practices to the detriment of what lies within that body, which often dictates the body's reactions and shapes its illnesses and stresses. And the Chinese medical world, despite its millennia-long acceptance of quite different medical principles, rather tamely followed where the West led, discarding much that had gone before, judging it to be unscientific and outmoded.

In the past 50 years or more, though, there has taken place a gradual tilting of the understanding of China's traditional medicine back towards greater respect for its past medical heritage, and a re-appraisal as to where it should be positioned in relation to Western medicine. Perhaps surprisingly, most of the impetus for this has come from Western traditional practitioners. And this is where I have come to understand that my arrival in China, bearing with me great respect for the validity of traditional Chinese medicine as shown in my practice of five element acupuncture, has allowed a breath of fresh air into the rather rigid, airless atmosphere in which its traditional acupuncture has been viewed and practised in its homeland. Perhaps because in England there has always been an oddly open acceptance of alternative medical practices, such as homeopathy, long practised by royalty, it was no coincidence that traditional Chinese acupuncture should have found such a welcome here when those first pioneers helped introduce it to this country some 50 years or more ago. And it was allowed to flourish in an atmosphere initially so blessedly free of the rigid educational framework enclosing much Western medicine, so that by falling to some extent off the Western medical radar it escaped much that might have hindered its development and practice, unlike what happened in China. In the UK to start with it was allowed to grow freely and flourish without the iron hand of state intervention hovering over it. Sadly, though, this freedom has gradually been eroded over recent years, once acupuncture moved into the sights of state-sponsored medicine, and there raised alarm bells. There were fears about the alien nature of its concepts, its denial of the need to obtain scientific proof for all that it did, and above all because of its undoubted, and therefore troubling, successes, vouched for by the many patients' feet now passing through acupuncturists' clinics.

The reactions of the Western medical world to what they often regarded as the invasion of dangerous practices into their highly controlled world led to the gradual introduction of more rigid requirements imposed upon acupuncture training institutes, and the increasing demand for degree-type courses with their emphasis, not on practical, vocational skills, so absolutely essential for an acupuncturist, but on the more intellectual exercises of written work and research projects. I realise now how fortunate I was to have slipped into my acupuncture training almost as one of the last students to benefit from so much freer an approach to our learning.

When I look back at my own progress from the lowest rungs of the acupuncture world as a student to where I am now, some 35 years later, I realise that the story of this journey into acupuncture has in some way mirrored the developments in the medical worlds of both the UK (and the West in general) and China. Certainly if you had asked me on that first evening at a party in London where I first encountered acupuncture in general, and five element acupuncture in particular, there would then have been no way at all that I could have predicted any of the profound changes to my life that that first, almost fortuitous encounter set in train. The changes in myself between the person I was then and the person I am now have been profound and, thankfully, totally life-affirming.

OTHER BOOKS IN THE FIVE ELEMENT ACUPUNCTURE SERIES

Blogging a Five Element Life

Nora Franglen
Paperback: £12.99/$19.95
ISBN: 978 1 84819 371 0
eISBN: 978 0 85701 328 6
248 pages

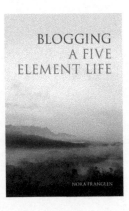

Based on her widely read blog, this collection includes Nora Franglen's reflections on her own continually developing five element practice, and the lived world between 2014 and March 2017, a time of enormous change.

Covering everything from politics, to her penchant for coffee shops, to how to treat patients effectively, and from tips on using moxa sticks to her acerbic thoughts on the effects of technology on society, Nora illustrates how the five elements influence, illuminate and enrich all aspects of her life, and vice versa.

On Being a Five Element Acupuncturist

Nora Franglen
Paperback: £12.99/$19.95
ISBN: 978 1 84819 236 2
eISBN: 978 0 85701 183 1
296 pages

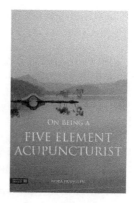

What does it mean to 'be' an acupuncturist? How does a highly experienced acupuncturist view her practice, her patients, and the world in general?

Based on her widely-read blog about the wholeness of life as a Five Element practitioner, Nora Franglen's breadth of interest shows how the curiosity and life experiences of the individual lie at the heart of what makes a true acupuncturist, over and beyond the necessary knowledge and expertise in the technicalities of practice. From her penchant for coffee shops to reflections on challenges she has experienced in the clinic, Nora illustrates how the Five Elements influence, illuminate and, ultimately, enrich all aspects of her life, and vice versa.

The Handbook of Five Element Practice

Nora Franglen
Paperback: £27.99/$45.00
ISBN: 978 1 84819 188 4
eISBN: 978 0 85701 145 9
184 pages

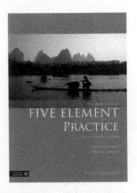

A practical companion for students and practitioners of five element acupuncture that helps stimulate thoughts, refresh memories and strengthen the foundation of practice.

With detailed outlines of the different components of five element diagnosis and treatment and overviews of the main characteristics of the five elements, this complete manual will support and invigorate practice. Full of examples, it explores the skills and techniques needed to nurture patient-practitioner relationships, assess patients correctly, select appropriate treatments and needle the points effectively. The book also includes a Teach Yourself Manual to further refresh understanding of this ancient form of healing.

This comprehensive handbook will be of immeasurable use to students and practitioners of five element acupuncture, as well as those who are interested in studying acupuncture and want to know more.